FRAMING THE MORON

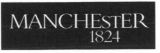

MANCHESTER
1824

Manchester University Press

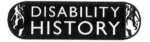

Series editors
Dr Julie Anderson, Professor Walton Schalick, III

This new series published by Manchester University Press responds to the growing interest in disability as a discipline worthy of historical research. The series has a broad international historical remit, encompassing issues that include class, race, gender, age, war, medical treatment, professionalisation, environments, work, institutions and cultural and social aspects of disablement including representations of disabled people in literature, film, art and the media.

Already published
Deafness, community and culture in Britain: leisure and cohesion, 1945–1995
Martin Atherton
Worth saving: disabled children during the Second World War
Sue Wheatcroft

FRAMING THE MORON

THE SOCIAL CONSTRUCTION OF FEEBLE-MINDEDNESS IN THE AMERICAN EUGENIC ERA

Gerald V. O'Brien

Manchester University Press

Published by Manchester University Press
Altrincham Street, Manchester M1 7JA, UK
www.manchesteruniversitypress.co.uk

British Library Cataloguing-in-Publication Data is available

Library of Congress Cataloging-in-Publication Data is available

ISBN 978 1 7849 9107 4 *paperback*

First published by Manchester University Press in hardback 2013

This edition first published 2016

The publisher has no responsibility for the persistence or accuracy of URLs for any external or third-party internet websites referred to in this book, and does not guarantee that any content on such websites is, or will remain, accurate or appropriate.

Printed by Lightning Source

Dedicated with love to my wife Jean,
and my children, Kevin, Mark, and Shannon.

Contents

Acknowledgements   ix
Introduction   1

1   Metaphors and the dehumanization of marginalized groups   18
2   The organism metaphor: the moron as a diseased entity   29
3   The animal metaphor: the moron as an atavistic subhuman   54
4   The war and natural catastrophe metaphors: the moron as an
    enemy force   82
5   The religious and altruistic metaphors: the moron as an immoral
    sinner and an object of protection   105
6   The object metaphor: the moron as a poorly functioning human   132
7   Conclusion   159

Bibliography   174
Index   197

Acknowledgements

I would first like to acknowledge those authors who spurred my interest in the topics of eugenics and metaphor analysis, and thus were influential in the direction of my research and eventual completion of this book. This list includes the late Steven Jay Gould and Burton Blatt, along with J. David Smith, Robert Proctor, Wolf Wolfensberger, Sam Keen, and George Lakoff. I would especially like to thank Jim Trent, who served as an important mentor for me, and whose own writings on the history of intellectual disability in the United States have been a great source of inspiration.

In July 2004 I was invited to attend a month-long institute on eugenics and disabilities in Germany, during which time our small group of scholars visited three of the six T–4 'euthanasia' locations. This institute was an extraordinary learning experience, and I thank the other participants for sharing it with me. I especially want to mention Sharon Snyder and David Mitchell for organizing the program, the Einstein Forum in Potsdam for supporting it, and the Deutscher Akademischer Austauch Dienst (DAAD) for providing me with a scholarship to attend. I'm also appreciative of the staffs at the Bernberg and Hadamar sites, as well as the many scholars who shared their expertise with us during our visit. Thanks also to all the wonderful people I've had the pleasure to meet over the years through the Society for Disability Studies (SDS).

My professional experiences in social work have been primarily in agencies serving persons with developmental disabilities, and my clients and colleagues served as an on-going source of inspiration. In fact, I think this work evolved largely from my curiosity about the fundamental difference between my pre-existing presumptions of persons with developmental disabilities and my actual experiences with such persons. I offer a debt of thanks to all my former clients and co-workers at the St Louis ARC, Community and Employment Services in Troy, Missouri, and the Springfield Developmental Center in Springfield, Illinois. Thanks especially to Amy Vazquez, Irv Rudasill, Kathy Meath, Darla Gamble, Tom Woolscy, and Cathy Barnett.

I was able to complete this book in part because of a sabbatical provided by Southern Illinois University, Edwardsville. I thank all those in the Department of Social Work, College of Arts and Sciences, and University who supported my work over the many years it took to see completion of the project, especially the late Tom Regulus, along with Kent Neely and Sharon Haas. More recently Vaughn Vandegrift, the University Chancellor, Al Romero, the Dean of the College of Arts and Sciences, and Larry Kreuger, the Chair of the

Department of Social Work, have been very supportive of my research. Thanks also to Steve Kerber in the University archives as well as all the other helpful staff at Lovejoy Library.

The following persons read portions of this manuscript at various stages of completion and provided valuable feedback; Jim Trent, Kathleen Tunney, and Duff Wrobbel. Thanks also to the following graduate assistants who helped me over the past decade or so by either tracking down or organizing resources, or by providing feedback on chapters: Christine Ellegood, Autumn Molinari, Mara Koerkenmeier, Michelle Maue, Melinda Brown, Megan Bundy, Emily Lane, Erin Steingruby, and Caroline Florczyk. Special thanks to Jana Leneave for devoting so much time to reviewing the book during my sabbatical semester. Thanks also to everyone at Manchester University Press, and especially to Emma Brennan and those who reviewed the book at various stages and made helpful suggestions for revisions. Versions of some content in this book were previously published in article form. These previous publications have been noted in the endnotes for the appropriate Chapter. I would like to thank these Journals for providing permission to use this material.

I especially want to express my deep gratitude to my family for their support over the course of this long project. Eugenics is, I admit, a very odd topic to be drawn toward, and both my immediate and my extended family have done a very good job of acting as if my chosen area of research is a perfectly reasonable use of my time and effort. My parents, Dan and Kay O'Brien, and my wife's parents, Don and Jackie McGurk, have been especially supportive. One of my few regrets about the project is that my father didn't live long enough to see the book in print. I also want to mention Fathers Tom Michel, Bob Gettinger, Tom O'Brien, and Jerry Kleba. In their lifelong commitments to social justice, and their belief in the dignity and value of all persons, they have been important sources of inspiration for me. Thanks also to my coach and mentor, the late Ron Jorgenson, for teaching me discipline and perseverance. These qualities served me well during the lengthy period of time I worked on this book.

Lastly, I can't adequately express my gratitude to my wife Jean for her ongoing support over the years. She has often put aside her own needs so that I could complete this work. By the time this book sees the light of day, I will have spent several decades, off and on, working on it. Someone who enjoys the pleasant things in life, Jean has had to spend way too much time over the past decade sharing the dark and disturbing spaces that this research has led me into. Also thanks to my children, Kevin, Mark, and Shannon for their continued love and support.

INTRODUCTION

Prior to laying out the remainder of this introduction, I want to first provide a brief explanatory note on terminology. I understand, of course, that many readers may be offended by the title of this book. As I try to explain later in this introduction as well as in the concluding chapter, there are several important reasons for the use of the term 'moron', as well as 'feeble-mindedness', both in the title and throughout the narrative. First, I believe historical works generally should employ the language of their time, for the sake of historical accuracy. The terms employed within this book were the professionally accepted diagnoses of the time. Secondly, a major theme of this work is the way in which words are introduced into language and 'filled up', if I might use the vessel metaphor discussed in Chapters 6 and 7. As I attempt to spell out within this book, the term 'moron' has an especially important role to play in the delineation of the targets of eugenic control, and indeed was created in large part for this particular purpose.

Over the past two decades, a rather large number of books focusing on the American eugenics movement have been published. These have covered virtually all aspects of the movement, including, for example, its antecedents and evolution, the major personalities involved, the relationship of American eugenics both to the Nazi race hygiene programs and contemporary genetic and bioethical developments and other aspects of the movement. This begs the relevant question: why another book on eugenics? My response to this is that this book is not 'on eugenics' in the sense that it is another overview of the movement and its effects. Rather, the primary objective of this book is to describe the various ways in which those in the movement 'framed' the concept of feeble-mindedness or moronity in order to justify the development of social control policies that would adversely impact the basic rights of a vast group of individuals who had committed no crimes.

The movement, therefore, serves as a point of departure from which readers can consider such metaphoric framings in a more universal sense. Indeed, as readers progress through Chapters 2–6, they will likely be struck by the parallels between past and present depictions of devalued groups and the social issues that relate to them. The dehumanization that was part and parcel of the eugenics movement did not occur in a vacuum, but is, I believe, best viewed when juxtaposed against similar social movements that sought to both diminish public regard for and limit the constitutional rights of a group of marginalized and vulnerable persons.[1] The term 'marginalized' refers simply to a disempowered stigmatized group on whom public antipathy may be projected, especially in times of high tension or mass anxiety. In a very real sense these persons live on the margins of society, so much so that they remain likely targets for removal from the community altogether. In some cases, as with the 'moron' class or presumed communist sympathizers, the target group may be very nebulous. The uncertainty of diagnosing exactly who falls within the group may both heighten anxiety related to its presumed members and allow advocates of control a great deal of latitude in describing and identifying the boundaries of the class.

'Alarm' movements such as that of the eugenic era, which seek to control a specific sub-group of the population because of a pervasive fear that is supposedly engendered by its members, are too often viewed in a highly simplistic manner. It is easy to contend, for example, that Japanese internment occurred because of the anger that accompanied Pearl Harbor, along with what might be construed to be somewhat reasonable concerns about the number of Japanese living in 'sensitive' areas of the West Coast of the United States. This contention, however, is largely dismissive of the decades of anti-Japanese sentiment, especially in California, that predated the internment decision, as well as of the fact that many Californians had a vested economic interest in removal of the Japanese. At times the fear of a rapidly expansive group of 'non-assimilable' Japanese approached a public panic, even long before the rise of the Axis powers.[2]

Eugenics is often discussed as a cautionary tale: an example of unchecked hysteria and pseudo-science run amok. This perception of the movement, however, is only partly accurate. The truth is that the presumptions and goals that supported eugenics have a very long history, and remain with us in somewhat altered versions today. The term 'eugenics' itself has taken on a highly pejorative connotation, and thus is differentially employed by writers on the basis of their personal or political positions. This can especially be seen in the presumptive relevance of eugenics within the context of current, as well as proposed, genetic research. Those calling for controls on such research use the term frequently, and, in addition, often allude to Nazi Germany as a relevant point of comparison for such research. Supporters of genetic innovations, however, frequently contend that eugenics is a remnant of the past, and that the substantive differences between historical and contemporary genetic policies and proposals make virtually all such analogies inaccurate and the result of simple fear-mongering. As is usually the case when such controversies arise, both views are partially correct.

The subject is important to introduce here, however, because such debates color our reaction to the term 'eugenics'. Readers of my age group, who grew up in the 1960s and 1970s, most likely never even knew of the term until fairly recently in their lives. I believe most of our children will be familiar with it by the time they finish high school, and our grandchildren at an even earlier age. These generations will mature in an age of genetic advancements that we could only dream or, depending on one's perspective, have nightmares about. Ethicists and policymakers will deliberate about the very essence of humanity, the nature of disability, and our role in determining the course of human evolution. It is important, therefore, before proceeding, to have a basic understanding of what is meant by eugenics.

At its most basic, the term 'eugenics', which was created by the Englishman Francis Galton, means 'good stock'.[3] As a means of carrying animal and plant breeding into the realm of human reproduction, eugenic policies can include any measures designed to ensure that the 'best' members of a society reproduce in greater numbers, or that the reproductive opportunities of the 'worst' members are limited, either voluntarily or, more often, by force. Important here is a widespread agreement within the culture of what constitutes the 'best' and 'worst' groups. One of the few universal certainties regarding eugenics as it has taken place in disparate cultures at different times is that those who support programs of controlled breeding seem assured that they themselves (along with their circle of family and acquaintances) stand firmly in the 'best' category.

Once one moves beyond this most basic premise, that certain qualities can be bred in humans just as in animal husbandry, problems arise. As Marouf Hasian wrote in his book *The Rhetoric of Eugenics in Anglo-American Thought*, eugenics can mean many things to different people. Most of the advocates of eugenics did hold a few core beliefs in common. For example, the belief that morons were a pressing social problem, and that sterilization and forced institutionalization should therefore be principal goals of the movement, was almost universally accepted by eugenicists in the United States as well as in Nazi Germany. However, as the authors of most secondary books on eugenics rightly point out, it would be inaccurate to therefore fall victim to the premise

that the movement was driven by a largely homogenous cadre of professionals, or even that the term 'eugenics' was understood in a similar way by the
majority of the movement's supporters. Hasain writes that '"eugenics" was
an ambiguous term that allowed many respectable Anglo-Americans to voice
their concerns on a number of social issues'.[4]

Those who came together in the United States to promote eugenic solu-
tions during the alarm era varied widely in their rationales for support, their
political philosophy, and what they considered the principal goals of the
program should be. Individual supporters could be referred to as falling into
one or more of the following categories: birth control supporters, religious
conservatives, progressive reformers, social Darwinists, virulent racists, activ-
ist feminists, public health advocates, persons who exploited the movement
for personal, professional, or financial gain, liberal-minded religious leaders,
curious scientists, and kindly philanthropists. This, moreover, is neither an
exhaustive nor a mutually exclusive list. Additionally, many of those who supported the movement did so for only a limited time, eventually falling away
from it for a variety of reasons. In Germany too, prior to Hitler's chancellor-
ship, there was no shared understanding among those various groups that supported eugenics either about how eugenic measures should be implemented
or about whether there was a high degree of overlap between 'race hygiene'
(especially in relation to Jews) and eugenic goals.[5]

Issues related to the description or goals of eugenics also need to be considered within the historical context that gave rise to interest in the subject in
the first place. As with other large-scale social movements, a confluence of professional, scientific, financial, political and ideological factors came together
during the first quarter of the twentieth century to support eugenic proposals
as a feasible means of adapting to societal transformations and perceived fears
(e.g., related to urbanization and immigration, women's rights, industrializa-
tion and technological development). As discussed in the following chapters,
but especially Chapter 4, eugenic interests were primarily stoked by dystopian
rather than utopian considerations. Writers on eugenics consistently warned
of the coming degeneration of the country that only their proposals would
forestall. This was in contrast to Nazi eugenics, where programs to encourage (or require) breeding among the desired segment of the population were
implemented alongside efforts to regulate the reproduction of those who were
deemed 'unfit'.

Common generalized assumptions of the movement's leaders and
supporters – that they all, for example, were mean-spirited elitists and bigots –
therefore constitute a vast oversimplification. The purpose of this book is not
to add fuel to the flames, and tarnish the reputations of long-dead individuals.

My intent is to consider the words and images that were employed to support eugenic goals, and analyze the role of these themes in the framing of marginalized groups, especially persons described as 'feeble-minded'. Along these lines, when I use the term 'eugenicist' in the book, which I naturally must do extensively, readers are to understand that not all of those who counted themselves as supporters of the movement necessarily agreed with each particular statement or recommendation attributed to the group as a whole. I have attempted to qualify these statements in cases where this is important. The question of how we define eugenics is taken up again in Chapter 7, where I consider the relationship between the early twentieth-century movement and current genetic and bioethical concerns.

The ambiguous meanings of the terms 'eugenics' and 'eugenicists' have been a principal reason for the confusion that has existed among secondary authors in describing not only the evolution of the movement, but also its decline in the United States. While many of these authors described the movement in the United States as ending during the 1930s, certain aspects of the era continued. Indeed, eugenic measures such as sterilization and institutionalization actually increased during this decade. It is true that the alarm period ended. However, while the widespread fear of a rapidly expanding feeble-minded population taking over the country diminished greatly following World War I, many aspects of eugenics continued unabated. In other words, it is most accurate to say that the rationales driving eugenic thinking changed during this time. I would refer readers to Wendy Kline's *Building a Better Race* for an insightful discussion of this issue.[6]

A final consideration in regard to the definition of eugenics, which also pertains to those bio-technologies which may be referred to as encompassing 'new eugenics', is that it could be argued that not all of the practices that are often said to be 'eugenic' rightly fall under this rubric, especially when we take into account the historical importance of heredity and family bloodlines in defining what constitutes a 'eugenic' practice. Many of those who were targeted for extermination by the Nazi euthanasia program, for example, were not likely to procreate. Either they had already been sterilized and/or institutionalized, or the extent of their disability precluded the likely possibility of reproduction. Even for those who might not have been sterilized, the cost of transporting them to the asylums and killing them far outweighed the cost of sterilization, which would have been just as effective from a purely eugenic standpoint. I would contend that the principal goal of the program was therefore not 'eugenic' since it was not simply to ensure that the bloodline of these persons was stopped, but rather to remove them from the world altogether. Likewise, one could argue that physician-assisted suicide or the aborting of a fetus with Tay-Sachs disease do not relate to eugenics per se, since those who would likely fall under such policies would not be expected to reproduce offspring. Many experts would consider this restriction of the word to be splitting hairs, but, like any term, 'eugenics' is at risk of losing any real meaning if it is expanded to an untoward degree. This is especially true in this case since we are dealing with a term that carries with it an extraordinary amount of emotional baggage, and is frequently exploited and misused for political and ideological purposes.[7]

There are a few additional notes on terminology. First, I have elected to utilize the terminology of the time almost exclusively in describing persons with intellectual disabilities[8] and other disability conditions. These terms, 'moron', 'imbecile', 'idiot', and 'feeble-minded', are certainly pejorative today, but were the accepted medical designations of the time. It is especially important that I employ the term 'moron', as this was a newly created designation at the beginning of the twentieth century, and how the term itself was framed, or the meaning it came to have, is a central element of this book.[9] James Trent wrote that by 'the First World War, the image of feeble minds created by professionals in the previous decades had shifted to a view of mental defectives that unlike previous views began to penetrate American consciousness. More than a shift of labels, the new term suggested new meaning and the necessity for a new social response.'[10] Additionally, since the word was a novel one that came with no 'conceptual baggage', this allowed supporters of eugenic control to fashion it in a way that served their interests. As Kline noted, "The construction and promotion of this 'high-grade moron' took on almost mythic proportions in the early twentieth century, adding to the appeal and authority of the eugenics movement."[11]

Other descriptors, such as 'degenerate' and 'defective', are also included in the book, since these were frequently invoked in eugenic writings. Such terms were even more imprecise than the term 'moron' and allowed eugenicists to expand the target group to include an even larger collection of devalued persons, including those who acted in presumably 'immoral' fashion but did not demonstrate a low level of intelligence. As the movement evolved, however, it became clear that such designations were unacceptably vague, and the more specific terms ('moron' and 'feeble-minded') were used with increasing frequency. I had originally intended to qualify these various terms by writing them as 'moron', 'degenerate', 'defective', and so on in the body of the book. In the end, however, I felt that this interrupted the flow of narrative, and I simply included them as they are, with the assumption that readers will understand that these terms are being used not because they were in any way accurate diagnostic categories but rather to provide a flavor of the original terminology.

Because so many other books have already been published related to the eugenics movement in the United States, this work does not provide an extensive historical overview. Readers who desire to know more about various aspects of the movement are referred to these previous publications, as I have attempted to delineate many of the seminal works in the footnotes. Since some readers, however, may have little awareness of the history of the movement, a very superficial historical introduction in provided here. Some of the more important elements of the movement are discussed further in Chapters 2–6.

Eugenics in the United States: a very brief history

With roots in the nineteenth century, the eugenics movement emerged as a major social force in the United States following the 1900 rediscovery of Mendel's laws of inheritance.[12] Based largely on the writings of England's Sir Francis Galton, the movement held that the human species could be improved through the systematic control of breeding practices.[13] Many of the early supporters of eugenics noted that the gains that had been made through the planned breeding of non-human animals should be carried over to the human species. If, as with these other animals, nations could develop methods to ensure that those with desired characteristics bred in greater numbers (a principle termed 'positive eugenics') while at the same time diminishing the breeding of those with undesirable characteristics (termed 'negative eugenics'), the species would presumably be improved. A similar term, 'euthenics', related to efforts to improve the species through environmental manipulation. Some eugenicists supported euthenics as a support for eugenic policy, but most believed that because of the hereditary deficits of morons and other target group members, neither they nor their progeny could be improved simply through education or an improved environment.

In the United States, early eugenics was inextricably connected to care and treatment of disabled persons, and especially those who were diagnosed as 'feeble-minded'.[14] Importantly, the development of the intelligence test shortly after the turn of the century allowed for the supposedly scientific delineation of the feeble-minded element of the population.[15] These persons, and especially the higher-functioning morons, were believed to be the nucleus from which a wide range of social evils, including poverty, drunkenness, sexually transmitted diseases, and a range of other disability conditions, emanated.[16] Eugenic concerns about these individuals were heightened by the eugenic family studies, a series of genealogical works that purported to describe the widespread dissemination of deleterious 'inherited' traits within specific families. The Juke, Kallikak, and other studies seemed to demonstrate that the contention of eugenicists about the hereditary nature of bad genetic traits was indeed valid.[17] In 1910 the Eugenics Record Office at Cold Springs Harbor, New York, was founded. Headed by Charles Davenport and Harry Laughlin, the leaders of the American movement, the Eugenics Record Office would become the center for eugenic propaganda and research during the movement.[18]

The primary methods of eugenic control included forced institutionalization and involuntary sterilization.[19] Following the turn of the century, institutional development flourished, pushed forward by the dissemination of propaganda that focused attention on the growing 'menace of the feeble-minded'. The placement of morons in segregated institutions, eugenicists said, would forestall their procreative opportunities.[20] Some supporters of 'sexual segregation' even suggested that presumably feeble-minded individuals (especially females of child-bearing age) should be forcibly institutionalized unless their care-givers could assure they would not reproduce.[21]

Many advocates of eugenics favored sterilization as a method of control, in part because it was more economically feasible than institutionalization.[22] During the first quarter of the century, tens of thousands of persons who were diagnosed as feeble-minded or insane would be institutionalized and/or sterilized for eugenic purposes. The most important eugenic legal victory came with the United States Supreme Court's *Buck v. Bell* decision in 1927, which allowed the states to practice involuntary sterilization.[23] An important aspect of social welfare history is that, in states such as Virginia and North Carolina, eugenic sterilization of persons labeled as having mental or intellectual disabilities paved the way for the forced sterilization of women (especially those from minority populations) receiving public assistance. Moreover, in some southern states eugenic arguments were also employed to support anti-miscegenation laws.[24]

A number of states additionally passed legislation restricting the ability of persons with feeble-mindedness and other disabilities to marry,[25] while other eugenicists called for the creation of public (e.g., tax-based) or private incentives that would either encourage the 'fit' to breed or discourage procreation among the 'unfit' segment of the population.[26] Many early supporters of birth control, including Margaret Sanger, also touted this as a potential method of eugenic control.[27] Some American eugenicists were also involved in the immigration restriction debate. In presenting pseudo-scientific data that seemed to demonstrate that many of the newer immigrants into the country were mentally or physically disabled, eugenicists played an important role in supporting the xenophobia that swept the United States following World War I. Important eugenicists such as Harry Laughlin were instrumental in supporting the development of the restrictive immigration acts of 1921 and 1924, which severely limited the number of immigrants allowed into the country.[28]

While the American movement would live on beyond the Great Depression, the hysterical fear of the moron, which had been its central driving force, lost impetus between 1915 and 1930. Institutional administrators and others came to admit that many cases of moronity were not genetic,[29] that most persons diagnosed as feeble-minded did not have large numbers of children,[30] and that cultural factors such as poverty and a lack of educational opportunities put many persons at risk for a diagnosis of feeble-mindedness.[31] Additionally, intelligence tests were called into question, especially as presumably 'normal' persons increasingly came to be diagnosed as morons.[32]

Importantly, while the eugenic fear of the moron was primarily stoked by professionals, including physicians, psychologists, institutional administrators, public health authorities, social workers, and zoologists and other scientists, as the movement progressed it became increasingly a part of popular culture. To some degree this was due to the efforts of eugenic organs such as the American Eugenics Society to integrate eugenic thinking into the mainstream of American life. As Susan Currell and Christina Cogdell describe in the selections that are included in their edited book *Popular Eugenics*, it was also supported by the expanded focus during the Progressive era in 'self-improvement', 'better living', and physical fitness, as well as early sex education literature.[33] While the early feminist and birth control movements held that sexuality should not be a source of shame and mystery, and that education regarding sexual development and decision-making were important elements of a progressive society, the flip side to this was that sexuality was becoming more of a 'public' interest, and could therefore perhaps be controlled by the community at large or policy-makers. It is certainly not surprising that sexual freedom and a control of sexuality were forces at the same time. These were, moreover, not necessarily inconsistent ideals, if freedom was allowed for those who 'ought' to procreate, and control was exerted upon those who 'ought' to be childless. Margaret Sanger, for example, held to both ideals. She called for women to have increased access to education related to sexuality and its control, and believed that this would provide them with greater freedom, as it would allow them to plan their pregnancies better. At the same time, however, she believed that some persons, especially morons, were incapable of such control and that responsible others needed to exert such control.[34]

The social purity movement and its efforts to stamp out alcoholism and venereal disease, and the largely successful efforts of eugenicists to include eugenic readings in college curriculums,[35] also served to familiarize the general public with eugenic tenets. Eugenics came to be further popularized by the development of early motion pictures on the topic,[36] the development of 'Better Babies' and 'Fitter Families' contests at state and local fairs,[37] and the infusion of eugenic topics in the novels and other works of even the most famous Western writers (e.g., Wells, Du Bois, Eliot, Hemingway, Woolf, Yeats) of the period.[38] As English noted, 'eugenics in some form can (and often does) show up on almost anyone's ideological map between 1890 and 1940 … in the United States of the 1910s and 1920s, eugenics became so widely accepted that it might be considered the paradigmatic modern American discourse.'[39]

By the 1930s, the primary supporters of eugenics who remained active in the American movement were persons who believed that eugenic goals could be extended beyond targeting simply persons and families with 'degenerate' qualities, but could also diminish the percentage of what were considered to be lower 'race types' within the nation. They believed, following the early 'racial anthropologists' such as August de Gobineau and Houston Stewart Chamberlain,[40] that the various 'races' could be viewed along a hierarchical dimension, with greater value given to those belonging to presumably higher races.[41] They also believed that miscegenation was diminishing the vitality of the Nordic or Aryan race. This segment of the American movement, then, directly influenced German notions of eugenics, both before and during the Third Reich.[42]

While a eugenic faction had developed in Germany before Hitler's ascent to power, it had little success in policy formation. Indeed, influential German eugenicists looked with envy at the gains wrought by the American eugenicists, especially the state sterilization laws.[43] Hitler's own interest in eugenics was an integral component of his overall scheme of race hygiene, and was widely disseminated a decade before his rise to power throughout the pages of *Mein Kampf*. He wrote, for example, that;

> A prevention of the faculty and opportunity to procreate on the part of the physically degenerate and mentally sick, over the period of only six hundred years, would not only free humanity from an immeasurable misfortune, but would lead to a recovery which today seems scarcely conceivable.[44]

Hitler proposed that measures of both negative and positive eugenics be combined to reverse race suicide in Germany. He felt that the Aryan segment of the population would dramatically decrease its breeding owing to economic and other forms of competition from other racial groups. Within his first year in power, he instituted a sweeping eugenic sterilization law that was targeted at persons with mental and physical disabilities. This policy would put Germany in the forefront of the eugenics movement, and by the time the program had run its course approximately 400,000 German citizens would be forcibly sterilized.[45] The German medical community largely supported the policy, not only because those who failed to ally themselves with the Nazis jeopardized their own positions, but also because they could point to the United States as leading the way, and thus providing moral cover for their program.[46]

In 1939, with the onset of their attack on Poland that marked the beginning of World War II, the Hitler government covertly implemented its most horrendous policy to eradicate persons with disabilities from the Reich, the T-4 euthanasia program. While the Nazis had been discreetly bringing about the deaths of thousands of disabled persons in institutions over the previous years, the T-4 program instituted the assembly-line killing apparatus that would characterize the Holocaust. The timing of the program is important, as the Nazis realized that they could more easily get away with it during wartime than during peacetime.[47] Before their utilization at the Holocaust sites, gas chambers were first installed and 'perfected' in six mental institutions. Over the course of a four-year period, these facilities took in and murdered approximately 70,000 'disabled' persons from throughout Germany, with the vast majority of these being persons labeled as 'feeble-minded' or 'insane'. The program ended around 1942, and the institutional apparatus and employees were removed to the eastern territories to help carry out the Holocaust. The killing of persons with disabilities, however, would continue until the end of the war, although the Nazis would resort to their earlier forms of murder, such as starvation and poisoning.[48]

With the full realization of the extent of the Nazis' eugenic programs, controlled human breeding largely became a taboo subject matter for several decades. While there was a direct connection between the American and German eugenic programs, this had much more to do with the homogeneity of the membership of the American movement at the time than with the programs themselves. In other words, most moderate supporters of eugenics within the United States had come to disassociate themselves from the movement before 1930. It would be oversimplifying matters greatly to imply that eugenics meant the same thing in both nations. Among leading eugenicists in each country, however, the principal target group for eugenic control remained fundamentally the same: persons with mental and intellectual disabilities.

Book outline

The first chapter of this book delineates the role of metaphors in dehumanizing marginalized groups, especially within the context of social policy development. This chapter thus sets the stage for the analysis chapters to follow. It also describes the broader implications of this study for dehumanization in a more general sense. This chapter also briefly details the five dehumanization themes. Chapters 2 through 6 each take up one of the metaphor themes. Following a brief introduction to the role of the metaphor theme in relation to dehumanization, the primary component of each of these analysis chapters is a description of the employment of the metaphor within the context of eugenics rhetoric, principally for the purpose of describing the need to control moronity within the nation. While the primary topic of this work is the American eugenics movement, examples related to eugenics in other countries, especially Nazi Germany will be included at times, especially for comparison's sake.

The primary goal of the final chapter will be to discuss the important contemporary implications for this study. Here I will especially consider the place of historical eugenics – and the metaphoric framings described – in relation to current discussions related to genetics and bioethics. I will also discuss the significance of eugenics for our understanding of the nature of disability, and the place of persons with disability within American society. Other issues that will be briefly taken up in Chapter 7 include a delineation of the potential motivating factors that may have led to the use of specific metaphor themes during the eugenics movement, the particular reasons why eugenicists came to target the 'moron' for social control, and the more broad implications of this study for understanding the nature of dehumanization.

Notes

1 See N. Sanford and C. Comstock (eds.), *Sanctions for Evil* (San Francisco: Jossey-Bass, Inc., 1971).

2 See, for example, D.W. Ryder, 'The Japanese bugaboo', *American Mercury* 3 (September 1924), '"The typhoon" – A dramatization of the yellow peril', *Current Literature* 52 (1912), 567–73; S.J. Gulick, *The American Japanese Problem* (New York: Charles Scribner's Sons, 1914).

3 F. Galton, *Inquiries into Human Faculty and its Development* (New York: E.P. Dutton & Co., 1907), p. 17.

4 M.A. Hasian, Jr., *The Rhetoric of Eugenics in Anglo-American Thought* (Athens, GA: University of Georgia Press, 1996), p. 14.

5 M. Burleigh, *The Third Reich: A New History* (New York: Hill and Wang, 2000), p. 347.

6 W. Kline, *Building a Better Race: Gender, Sexuality and Eugenics from the Turn of the Century to the Baby Boom* (Berkeley: University of California Press, 2001), p. 19.

7 G.V. O'Brien, 'Eugenics, genetics and the minority group model of disabilities: Implications for social work advocacy', *Social Work* 56 (2011), 347–54.

8 Over the course of the last decade and a half or so, there has been widespread

debate in professional circles about nomenclature in relation to those who may be described as (among other terms) having mental retardation or being cognitively or intellectually disabled or developmentally disabled. I generally prefer the middle two terms, though all are preferable to 'intellectually challenged' and similar phrases.

9 One additional nomenclature note: while 'person first' language is generally (and for what I believe are valid reasons) employed in any contemporary scholarship pertaining to those with disabilities, I do not utilize it throughout the book. There are several reasons for this: first, especially in view of how often such terms are employed, it would be much too wordy, and secondly, the original terminology provides a much more accurate feel for the historical time that is described. When I refer to morons, imbeciles, etc., these socially constructed terms should be interpreted as 'persons who were labeled as morons or imbeciles'.

10 J.W. Trent, Jr., *Inventing the Feeble Mind: A History of Mental Retardation in the United States* (Berkeley: University of California Press, 1994), p. 141.

11 Kline, *Building a Better Race*, p. 19.

12 For examples of eugenic proposals prior to Galton, which go back to the ancient Greeks, see Plato, *The Republic*, trans. D. Lee, reprint edn. (Harmondsworth, Middlesex: Penguin Books, Ltd., 1986), pp. 240–1; J.O. Hertzler, *The History of Utopian Thought* (New York: Cooper Square Publishers, Inc., 1965); A.G. Roper, 'Ancient eugenics', *Mankind Quarterly* 32 (1992), 383–418; M.S. Iseman, *Race Suicide* (New York: Cosmopolitan Press, 1912). For Mendel's influence, see S.J. Gould, *The Mismeasure of Man* (New York: W.W. Norton and Co., 1981); C.N. Degler, *In Search of Human Nature* (New York: Oxford University Press, 1991); A.E. Klein, *Threads of Life: Genetics from Aristotle to D.N.A.* (Garden City, NJ: Natural History Press, 1970).

13 Galton's major writings related to eugenics include *Hereditary Genius* (New York: D. Appleton and Co., 1870), and *Inquiries into Human Faculty and its Development*. Later works such as 'Eugenics: Its definition, scope, and aims', *American Journal of Sociology* 10 (1904), 1–25 (discussion included), and the reprint of a 1909 collection of his shorter writings on the topic, entitled *Essays in Eugenics* (Washington, DC: Scott Townsend Publishers, 1996), also provide important information on the development of Galton's eugenic philosophy. For the life of Galton, see D.W. Forrest, *Francis Galton: The Life and Work of a Victorian Genius* (New York: Taplinger Publishing Co., Inc., 1974).

14 See, for example, G.V. O'Brien and M. Bundy, 'Reaching beyond the "moron": Eugenic control of secondary disability groups', *Journal of Sociology and Social Welfare* 36 (2009), 153–71; J.D. Smith, *Minds Made Feeble: The Myth and Legacy of the Kallikaks* (Austin, TX: Pro-Ed, 1985); Trent, *Inventing the Feeble Mind*. For an insightful account of the perception of feeble-mindedness in Britain, both before and during the eugenic era, see M. Jackson, *The Borderland of Imbecility: Medicine, Society and the Fabrication of the Feeble Mind in Late Victorian and Edwardian England* (Manchester: Manchester University Press, 2000).

15 For the intelligence tests, see C.C. Brigham, *A Study of American Intelligence* (London: Princeton University Press, 1923); P.H. DuBois, *A History of Psychological Testing* (Boston: Allyn and Bacon, Inc., 1970); R.E. Fancher, *The Intelligence Men: Makers of the I.Q. Controversy* (New York: W.W. Norton and Co., 1985); Gould, *The Mismeasure of Man*; L.J. Kamin, *The Science and Politics of I.Q.* (Potomac, MD: Lawrence Erlbaum Association, 1974). J. Peterson, *Early Conceptions and Tests of Intelligence* (Westport, CT: Greenwood Press, 1969).

16 See, for example, J.C. Carson, 'Prevention of feeble-mindedness from a moral and legal standpoint', in *Proceedings of the National Conference of Charities and Correction* (Boston: G.H. Ellis, 1898), pp. 294–303; H. MacMurchy, 'The relation of feeble-mindedness to other social problems', *Journal of Psycho-Asthenics* 21 (1916), 58–63.

17 The earliest of the family studies was that of the Jukes, and the most publicized during the eugenic era was that of the Kallikaks. See R.L. Dugdale, *The Jukes: A Study in Crime, Pauperism, Disease, and Heredity*, 4th edn. (New York: G.P. Putnam's Sons, 1910); H.H. Goddard, *The Kallikak Family* (New York: Arno Press, 1912). Also see M.S. Kostir, *The Family of Sam Sixty* (Mansfield, OH: Press of Ohio State Reformatory, 1916). The best overview and analysis of the studies as a whole is in N.H. Rafter's *White Trash: The Eugenic Family Studies 1877–1919* (Boston: Northeastern University Press, 1988). For more on Deborah Kallikak and the study that bore her name, see the various articles by Elizabeth S. Kite, 'Two brothers', *Survey* 27 (1912), 1861–4, 'Unto the third generation', *Survey* 28 (1912), 789–91, 'The "Piney's"', *Survey* 31 (1913), 9–13, 38–40, and 'Mental defect as found by the field-worker', *Journal of Psycho-Asthenics* 17 (1913), 145–54, along with Helen T. Reeves's 'The later years of a noted mental defective', *Journal of Psycho-Asthenics* 43 (1938), 194–200.

18 For information on the Eugenics Record Office, see D.J. Kevles, *In the Name of Eugenics* (New York: Alfred A. Knopf, 1985), or any of the other general works on the American movement referred to in this chapter. For primary sources, see the following writings by H.H. Laughlin: 'Report on the organization and the first eight months' work of the Eugenics Record Office', *American Breeders Magazine* 2:2 (1911), 107–12, 'An account of the work of the Eugenics Record Office', *American Breeders Magazine* 3:2 (1912), 119–23, and 'First Annual Conference of Eugenics Field Workers', *American Breeders Magazine* 3:4 (1912), 265–9.

19 For a description of the relative benefits of each, see Henry Goddard's 'Sterilization and segregation', *Indiana Bulletin* (December 1912), 424–8.

20 James Trent, in his book *Inventing the Feeble Mind*, provides a very good historical overview of the history of institutionalization of persons diagnosed as being feeble-minded.

21 See 'Feeble minded boys committed under new law', *Chicago Tribune* (19 November 1915), p. 5; *The Kallikaks of Kansas: Report of the Kansas Commission on Provision for the Feebleminded* (Topeka: Kansas State Printing Plant, 1919), p. 8;

W.E.W. Wallin, 'A program for the state care of the feeble minded and epileptic', *School and Society* 4 (11 November 1916), 723–31.

22 H.H. Laughlin, 'The eugenical sterilization of the feeble-minded', *Journal of Psycho-Asthenics* 31 (1925), 210–18. For the early history of sterilization procedures, see Paul Popenoe's 'The progress of eugenic sterilization', *Journal of Heredity* 25 (1934), 19–25. For a fascinating primary source, see F.H. Pilcher's 'Superintendent's report', in *Seventh Biennial Report of the Superintendent, Kansas Asylum for Idiotic and Imbecile Youth at Winfield* (Topeka: Press of the Hamilton Printing Company, 1894), pp. 7–8. Pilcher discusses the benefit of castration of institutionalized persons as a method of mitigating masturbation.

23 Philip R. Reilly provides a comprehensive overview of eugenic sterilization in *The Surgical Solution: A History of Involuntary Sterilization in the United States* (Baltimore: Johns Hopkins University Press, 1991). For the Carrie Buck case specifically, see J.D. Smith and K.R. Nelson's *The Sterilization of Carrie Buck* (Far Hills, NJ: New Horizon Press, 1989) or M. Dudziak's 'Oliver Wendell Holmes as a eugenic reformer: Rhetoric in the writing of constitutional law', *Iowa Law Review* 71 (1986), 833–67.

24 See, for example, E. Black, *War against the Weak: Eugenics and America's Campaign to Create a Master Race* (New York: Four Walls Eight Windows, 2003); P. Newbeck, *Virginia hasn't Always been for Lovers: Interracial Marriage Bans and the Case of Richard and Mildred Loving* (Carbondale, IL: Southern Illinois University Press, 2004); E.J. Larson, *Sex, Race and Science: Eugenics in the Deep South* (Baltimore: Johns Hopkins University Press, 1996), pp. 162–3; A.C. Kennedy, 'Eugenics, "degenerate girls", and social workers during the Progressive era', *Affilia: Journal of Women and Social Work* 23 (2008), 23–37; J. Paul, 'State eugenic sterilization history: A brief overview', in J. Robitscher (ed.), *Eugenic Sterilization* (Springfield, IL: Charles C. Thomas, 1973), pp. 25–40.

25 C.B. Davenport, 'Marriage laws and customs', in *Problems in Eugenics: Papers Communicated to the First International Eugenics Congress* (London: Eugenics Education Society, 1912), pp. 151–5.

26 See, for example, Rev. W.T. Sumner, 'The health certificate: A safeguard against vicious selection in marriage', in *Proceedings of the First National Conference on Race Betterment* (Battle Creek, MI: Race Betterment Foundation, 1914), pp. 509–12; H.L. Mencken, 'Utopia by sterilization', *American Mercury* 41 (1937), 399–408.

27 M. Sanger, 'Birth control and racial betterment', *Birth Control Review* 3:2 (1919), 11–12, and *The Pivot of Civilization* (New York: Brentano's Publishers, 1922). Many eugenicists were wary of birth control as an effective eugenic control method, as they believed that the more 'fit' parents would be the ones to primarily take advantage of such opportunities. See, for example, H.P. Fairchild, 'From dysgenic to eugenic birth control', *Birth Control Review* 2:7 (1935), 2–3; H.H. Laughlin, 'Further studies on the historical and legal development of eugenical sterilization in the United States', *Journal of Psycho-Asthenics* 41 (1936), 98.

28 See K. Calavita, *U.S. Immigration Law and the Control of Labor: 1820–1924*

(London: Academic Press, Inc., 1984), pp. 107–13; testimony of H.H. Laughlin, 8 March 1924, in *Europe as an Emigrant-Exporting Continent and the United States as an Immigrant Receiving Nation*, U.S. House of Representatives, Committee on Immigration and Naturalization, pp. 1231–318; Kamin, *The Science and Politics of I.Q.*; G.V. O'Brien, 'Indigestible food, conquering hordes, and waste materials: Metaphors of immigrants and the early immigration restriction debate in the U.S.', *Metaphor and Symbol* 18 (2003), 33–47.

29 T.S. Harding, 'Are we breeding weaklings?', *American Journal of Sociology* 42 (1936), 672–81.

30 I.W. Cox, 'The folly of human sterilization', *Scientific American* 151 (1934), 188–90.

31 A. Deutsch, *The Mentally Ill in America: A History of their Care and Treatment from Colonial Times* (Garden City, NY: Doubleday, Doran and Co., 1938); P.J. Ryan, '"Six blacks from home": Childhood, motherhood, and eugenics in America', *Journal of Policy History* 19 (2007), 253–81. Also see F. Boas, 'Instability of human types', G.W. Stocking, Jr. (ed.), *The Shaping of American Anthropology 1883–1911: A Franz Boas Reader* (New York: Basic Books, Inc., 1974), pp. 214–18.

32 Gould, *The Mismeasure of Man*; A. Scheinfeld, *You and Heredity* (New York: Frederick A Stokes Co., 1939), p. 219; Reilly, *The Surgical Solution*, p. 142.

33 S. Currell and C. Cogdell (eds.), *Popular Eugenics: National Efficiency and American Mass Culture in the 1930s* (Athens: Ohio University Press, 2006). For examples of 'eugenic' books that were directed at the general population, see W.J. Hadden, *The Science of Eugenics and Sex Life*, ed. C.H. Robinson, 2nd edn. (W.R. Vansant, 1914); B.G. Jefferis and J.L. Nichols, *Safe Counsel or Practical Eugenics*, 37th edn. (Naperville, IL: J.L. Nichols & Co., 1924); T.W. Shannon, *Nature's Secrets Revealed*, 3rd edn. (Marietta, OH: S.A. Mullikin Company, 1915).

34 Sanger, *The Pivot of Civilization*.

35 S. Selden, *Inheriting Shame: The Story of Eugenics and Racism in America* (New York: Teachers College, 1999).

36 M.S. Pernick, *The Black Stork: Eugenics and the Death of 'Defective' Babies in American Medicine and Motion Pictures since 1915* (New York: Oxford University Press, 1996).

37 R. Gilman, 'Better babies', in *Proceedings of the First National Conference on Race Betterment* (Battle Creek, MI: Race Betterment Foundation, 1914), pp. 272–8; W.F. Martin, 'Better babies contest', in *Proceedings of the First National Conference on Race Betterment* (Battle Creek, MI: Race Betterment Foundation, 1914), pp. 554–5; L.L. Lovett, '"Fitter families for future firesides": Florence Sherbon and popular eugenics', *Public Historian* 29:3 (2007), 69–85.

38 See the examples in L.A. Cuddy and C.M. Roche (eds.), *Evolution and Eugenics in American Literature and Culture, 1880–1940* (Lewisburg: Bucknell University Press, 2003); D.J. Childs, *Modernism and Eugenics: Woolf, Eliot, Yeats, and the Culture of Degeneration* (Cambridge: Cambridge University Press, 2001); B.L. Nies, *Eugenic Fantasies: Racial Ideology in the Literature and Popular Culture of*

the 1920's (New York: Routledge, 2002), and D.K. English, *Unnatural Selections: Eugenics in American Modernism and the Harlem Renaissance* (Chapel Hill: University of North Carolina Press, 2004).

39   English, *Unnatural Selections*, p. 2.

40   A. De Gobineau, *The Inequality of Human Races*, trans. A. Collins, reprint edn. (Los Angeles: Noontide Press, 1966); H.S. Chamberlain, *Foundations of the Nineteenth Century*, trans. J. Lees, reprint edn. (New York: John Lane Co., 1913).

41   Gould, *The Mismeasure of Man*; J.H. Landman, 'Race betterment by human sterilization', *Scientific American* 150 (1934), 293.

42   See S. Kühl, *The Nazi Connection: Eugenics, American Racism, and German National Socialism* (New York: Oxford University Press, 1994) and M.D. Miller, *Terminating the 'Socially Inadequate': The American Eugenicists and the German Race Hygienists, California to Cold Spring Harbor, Long Island to Germany* (Commack, NY: Malamud-Rose, Publisher, 1996). According to Edwin Black, several American eugenicists had even received letters from Adolf Hitler praising their works. He even called Madison Grant's influential *Passing of the Great Race* his 'Bible'. See Black, *War against the Weak*, p. 259.

43   Kühl, *The Nazi Connection*. For more on the relationship between the German and American programs, see P. Crook, 'American eugenics and the Nazis: Recent historiography', *European Legacy* 7 (2002), 363–81.

44   A. Hitler, *Mein Kampf*, trans. R. Manheim, reprint edn. (Boston: Houghton Mifflin Co., 1971), pp. 404–5.

45   'Eugenical sterilization in Germany', *Eugenical News* 18:5 (1933), 89–94; R.N. Proctor, *Racial Hygiene: Medicine under the Nazis* (Cambridge, MA: Harvard University Press, 1988). The reaction of those American eugenicists who continued to embrace eugenic control at this point was on the whole very supportive of the Nazi sterilization program. See, for example, C. Campbell, 'Praise for Nazis', *Time* (9 September 1935), 20–1; 'U.S. Eugenicist Hails Nazi Racial Policy', *New York Times* (29 August 1935), 5; L. Whitney, *The Case for Sterilization* (New York: Frederick A. Stokes Co., 1934), pp. 137–8; P. Popenoe, 'The German sterilization law', *Journal of Heredity* 25 (1934), 260.

46   'Case for sterilization', *Living Age* 357 (1939), 135–7.

47   M. Burleigh, *Death and Deliverance: 'Euthanasia' in Germany 1900–1945* (Cambridge: Cambridge University Press, 1994); P. Weindling, *Health, Race and German Politics between National Unification and Naziism, 1870–1945* (Cambridge: Cambridge University Press, 1989).

48   Burleigh, *Death and Deliverance*; B. Müller-Hill, *Murderous Science: Elimination by Scientific Selection of Jews, Gypsies and Others: Germany 1933–1945*, trans. G.R. Fraser (New York: Oxford University Press, 1988); Proctor, *Racial Hygiene*; W. Wolfensberger, 'The extermination of handicapped people in World War II Germany', *Mental Retardation* 19 (1981), 1–7.

METAPHORS AND THE DEHUMANIZATION OF MARGINALIZED GROUPS[1]

Why is one person, or animal, abused and not another? If this is under-stood, everything is understood. In the face of greatly mounting criticism, one Canadian official commented on the slaughter of 50,000 harp-seal pups each year in the Maritime Provinces: 'If we could find a way to make pup seals look like alligators, our problems would be over.' It was the job of Joseph Goebbels to make pup seals look like alligators and Jews and Poles look like subhumans.[2]

Metaphors, problem framing, and social policy

In his book *Dinosaur in a Haystack*, Steven Jay Gould tells of a visit to Greece, where his view of the Parthenon was briefly obscured by a moving van. His annoyance turned to amusement when he saw that the sign on the van read 'metaphora'. As a vehicle for changing the location of things ('meta') by moving or carrying them ('phor'), Gould noted, the van symbolized what a metaphor is.[3] Schon writes that '[m]etaphorical utterances' constitute the '"carrying over" of frames or perspectives from one domain of experience to another'.[4] At their most basic, linguistic metaphors include a source domain and a target domain. In the case of the 'Jew as bacillus' metaphor that was frequently employed by the Nazis, for example, the bacillus constitutes the source domain, the Jew the target. The primary rationale for the metaphor, then, is to 'carry over' or transfer important, though often covert, aspects of the source object or person onto the target.

Those who perceive metaphors simply as providing an interesting or pic-turesque mode of describing people and issues with little real impact fail to understand their importance.[5] Susan Sontag noted that metaphor use has existed for a very long time in human societies and has served as the 'spawning ground of most kinds of understanding, including scientific understanding, and expressiveness'.[6] To quote Steven Jay Gould, 'a scholar's choice of metaphor usually provides our best insight into the preferred modes of thought and surrounding social circumstances that so influence all human reasoning, even the scientific modes often viewed as fully objective in our mythology'.[7]

As many writers have noted, the use of metaphors is a principal way in which we comprehend the world around us, even if we seldom realize it. According to David Allbritton, the metaphoric connection of source and target domains can have a strong influence on how we come to perceive and thus respond to the latter. He added that a 'related cognitive function that metaphor often fulfills is that of providing a framework for understanding a new domain or for restructuring the understanding of a familiar domain'.[8] George Lakoff, the leading contemporary metaphor analyst and scholar in the United States, contended that '[a] large proportion of our most commonplace thoughts make use of an extensive, but unconscious, system of metaphorical concepts, that is, concepts from a typically concrete realm of thought that are used to comprehend another, completely different domain'.[9]

Metaphors may not only carry meaning about the alleged 'essence' of a thing, person, or group, but may also serve as a vehicle for communicating overt or underlying messages about the recommended modes of treating or responding to the target.[10] For example, the 'Jew as bacillus' metaphor obviously was useful to the Nazis since many of the aspects of a bacillus (potential for harm, spread, inconspicuousness invasion, etc.) served to aptly describe Nazi presumptions about Jews, especially those on their eastern border (e.g., Polish, Russian, and Hungarian Jews). Moreover, if Jews could be perceived as being like a bacillus that threatened anyone with whom they came into contact, their segregation from the rest of the community in ghettos, and later their 'disinfection' or mass killing, might be more easily accepted by Germans. As will be further described below, in the political arena selected policy responses underlie the employment of particular metaphoric patterns and 'framings' of social issues and marginalized groups.

In addition to drawing attention to linguistic metaphors, scholars frequently point out the importance of more broad 'conceptual metaphors'. Indeed, it is conceptual metaphors that are primarily described within the analysis section of this book. According to Allbritton, a conceptual metaphor relates not just to a metaphorical term or phrase, but to a general way of thinking about a particular object (or objects) or person (or persons).[11] To continue the above example, the general perception that arose in Nazi Germany that the Jews were a plague or disease was reinforced not only by linguistic metaphors such as 'the Jew is a bacillus', but also by numerous non-metaphorical arguments and actions, including 'quarantine' measures, questions about the physical health and cleanliness of Jews in eastern territories, a belief that the Jew's 'essence' could be transmitted to non-Jews and indeed could easily contaminate the Aryan gene pool, and the victimization of those who assisted or even simply communicated with Jews. German citizens realized that, for their own protection if for no other reason, they should treat Jews as if they carried a contagious disease. Even those persons who might have 'Jewish blood' but who identified themselves as Aryan were to be avoided, just as one might refrain from contact with an asymptomatic carrier of disease.

In addition to providing a general 'frame' against which the target is described, conceptual metaphors, Allbritton wrote, can influence the way in which information about the target 'is processed and represented in memory'.[12] In other words, additional knowledge about the group or event is considered in light of the existing conceptual metaphor. Once a particular conceptual metaphor is embraced as an apt way of viewing the target, it may be extremely difficult to replace it with a contrasting mode of framing the issue or group. De Vos and Suárez-Orozco contended that once we come to embrace 'feelings of social revulsion and disgust' toward a particular group of persons, it is extremely unlikely that newly acquired information that runs counter to this stereotypical image will be mentally processed in a way that allows us to engage in a marked readjustment of the original image.[13] In part this is due to the fact that metaphors often act subconsciously, impacting our feelings and actions in ways that we are not even aware of, and their effects are often long-lasting.

Metaphors and marginalization

The more closely we look, the more we realize that a select collection of pejorative rhetorical themes have been employed over time for the purpose of denigrating various marginalized community groups. Wolf Wolfensberger, the Syracuse University emeritus professor who introduced the concept of normalization into the United States, noted that '[w]hen we review history and literature, it becomes apparent that regardless of time or place, certain roles are particularly apt to be thrust upon deviant persons. The way in which these roles transcend time, distance and culture is remarkable.'[14] In the same vein Sam Keen wrote that '[w]hat we will find is that wars come and go, but – strangely, amid changing circumstances – the hostile imagination has a certain standard repertoire of images it uses to dehumanize the enemy'.[15] What Keen says of warfare is just as true in regard to the many forms of oppression that are rationalized by arguments of self-preservation, economic security, race or class stabilization, the augmentation of control, the protection of one's family, or paternalistic intent.

Metaphors and other rhetorical devices have frequently been employed as vehicles for fostering dehumanization,[16] influencing societal ideology and policy development, and providing justification for the extreme actions that are taken against 'deviant' or stigmatized groups. When persons or groups are consistently compared to a denigrated, distasteful, or threatening object, animal, person, or group, it is the intention of the speaker or writer that facets of the pejoratively viewed source domain become associated with the target domain, for the purpose of diminishing the value of the latter.[17] As Burton Blatt wrote, one of the principal ways 'to create monsters out of human beings' is to 'construct a story so as to make them into something they do not want to be'.[18]

In his book *Dehumanizing the Vulnerable: When Word Games Take Lives*, William Brennan describes some of the important themes that function as source domains. As Brennan writes, '[i]n many instances, the most significant factor determining how an object will be perceived is not the nature of the object itself, but the words employed to characterize it'.[19] Vitriolic language, he adds, often punctuated by metaphors, is a constituent feature of any major effort to dehumanize or oppress a marginalized segment of the population.[20] What he terms 'semantic warfare', Brennan adds, 'does not ordinarily burst upon the scene helter-skelter. It is not an accidental, spontaneous, or chaotic episode, but a deliberate and unremitting phenomenon usually undergirded by fully elaborated systems of concepts, beliefs, and myths.'[21] As a general rule, those who engage in violence or denigration, or advocate social control measures against others, do not want to be perceived as acting inhumanely or without compelling justification. Whenever, therefore, widespread efforts are made to control, disparage, or even exterminate stigmatized persons, various rationales are employed to portray the target group as a threat to society, a subhuman entity, or both.

The employment of disparaging metaphors as a means of describing an undesirable target group does more than simply present covert rationales for their possible control. Such metaphors also are a principal means by which those who want to expand their power or sphere of influence attempt to legitimize their role as definers of the group or of the social problem(s) targeted.[22] Lise Noël noted that '[b]efore being stripped of their property or rights, the oppressed are robbed of their identity.' 'The dominator', she continues, 'defines this identity in their stead, reducing it to a difference that is then labelled inferior.'[23]

As Michel Foucault, Erving Goffman, Thomas Szasz, and others have noted, in the medical field, as well as psychiatry and other professions that are marked by the labeling of human conditions by established experts or authority figures, such diagnosis, while it may benefit the 'patient' in certain ways, also reinforces the power relationship between the diagnosed person and the 'expert'.[24] Identifying the other is not only an important means of attempting to exert power, but may even carry with it presumptions of property rights. Many cottage industries have developed and numerous job opportunities have arisen as an outgrowth of expanded diagnostic 'expertise' and the subsequent reification of vague disability and medical and psychological conditions.

Efforts by marginalized community groups to reestablish their own identity in society are therefore a central theme in contemporary scholarship on prejudice and discrimination. Much of the current writing in disability studies, for example, deals with this issue. Some persons with a disability, such as many individuals who are deaf, do not even consider themselves disabled, and resent efforts by others to define them that way. Even many persons who self-identify as disabled do not necessarily consider their disability to be their primary identifying attribute, even if others consider it so. Additionally, in cases where persons do identify their disability as a core feature of their identity, the meaning that the condition has is often very different from that which observers assume, especially since many non-disabled persons tend to 'awfulize' disabilities and see only their negative consequences.[25]

Identifying the target group as deviant or apart from the norm is also a means of affirming the 'foundational values' of the prevailing status quo, or of reinforcing expected normative behavior.[26] Identifying community subgroups as outside the societal mainstream or as rejecting cultural norms or values is a means of supporting the image of entrenched powers as being inherently superior to such groups. It also serves to foster 'victim-blaming' whereupon the oppression of such individuals is perceived as due to their own inadequacies or inappropriate decisions. Therefore, writes Noël, once the members of marginalized groups 'embark on the path toward rejection of their alienation, the challenge for the oppressed is to expose the relativity of the various identities and the subjective foundations of the judgments determining social hierarchies'.[27]

The sociopolitical implications of derisive metaphors

Since both linguistic and conceptual metaphors are frequently employed to 'frame' a social problem or group in a way that is desired by the majority or important stakeholders, they have a great deal of influence in the policy arena. The significance of such perceptual frames, for example, can easily be gauged by perusing the United States *Congressional Record* when a controversial issue or proposed policy is discussed, especially when a degree of social control or diminution of individual rights is a potential policy solution. Such discussions are often laced with picturesque terminology and potent metaphors to further a specific 'image' of the problem.[28] To quote George Lakoff: '[b]ecause so much of our social and political reasoning makes use of this system of metaphorical concepts, any adequate appreciation of even the most mundane social and political thought requires an understanding of this system'.[29]

As Donald Schön wrote, problem-setting, or the extension of a particular view of a social problem, is just as important in policymaking, than problem-solving, if not more important. Particular framings of social issues that serve the interests of economic or political stakeholder groups often depend 'upon metaphors underlying the stories which generate problem setting and set the directions of problem solving'.[30] Another benefit of metaphor use within the policy arena, Schön added, is that they may vastly simplify very complex situations.[31] The decision to wage a war, for example, is normally the end result of an extraordinarily complicated series of events and personal, institutional, resource, and international relationships. When the decision is made, however, those in power will need to gain the support of the public, or at least alienate the opposition. In addition to supplying presumably rational explanations for the decision, they will invoke a host of metaphors to vilify the enemy and present the battle as a necessary means of self-preservation. A successful rhetorical campaign in support of war will isolate those who do not support it as weak, impassive, fence-sitting, milque-toast lackeys of the enemy whose treasonous questioning of the decision is even putting their own families at risk.

Metaphors are often employed also to stereotype or to generalize particular examples as being illustrative of the entire group in question. Consider, for example, the 1996 United States welfare reform legislation, the Personal Responsibility and Work Opportunity Reconciliation Act. This law was passed, in large measure, because of public disgust about 'welfare as we know it'. A great deal of public pressure was exerted on legislators to support the policy. The question then arises: what was the source of this public anger? Was it the result of reasoned public discourse and a rational collective deliberation of the factual information and objective research studies related to the impact of various 'welfare' programs or demographic trends? Or did the perception that welfare recipients were ungrateful, lazy 'parasites' who lived off the public dole while contributing nothing in return become the dominant, indeed virtually the only, way in which the issue was viewed? The perception of the target group, formed in large part by a conceptual metaphor (person as parasite), forced the change. Indeed, the perception that welfare recipients[32] are persons who need to become responsible can be seen in the title of the legislation ('personal responsibility').

As the ethicist George Annas noted in his article on metaphors and the United States health care system, policy decisions are closely related to the way in which we think about an issue (such as health care delivery) vis-à-vis metaphors. Annas writes that an issue can be reframed and viewed from a different perspective if a varying metaphor theme is employed to describe it, and if this alternate framing is widely accepted as a reasonable way of viewing the issue.[33] As noted above, however, this is not necessarily an easy task, especially if the prevailing metaphors have taken hold. As Lakoff demonstrated, those policymakers who are best able to utilize conceptual metaphors in framing issues are the most apt to garner public support for their positions.[34]

Metaphors are an important component of the policy process not only because they can identify the way in which important stakeholders believe problems 'should' be viewed, and thus the proper policy response(s). They also provide a potent means of evoking 'strong emotional responses in listeners'. As noted above, many metaphors are effective on a subconscious level and, especially when the goal is to denigrate a marginalized group, tie into powerful inherent aversions, such as our fear of bodily invasion (by a parasite, germ, virus, poison, etc.), safety concerns and the need to act as protectors for our children; latent gender constructs (e.g., for males, strength, action, independence, and for females, beauty, nurturance, romance); and various manifestations of disgust or repugnance.[35] As Levin wrote, a principal attribute of alarm movements, and the rhetoric that fuels them, is that they 'excite deep unconscious wishes and anxieties and tap primitive and infantile ways of thinking.'[36]

Alarm movements such as that of the eugenic era, wherein the social control of a specific subgroup or closely aligned subgroups of the population is called for as a means of restabilizing society, are important not only because they involve a passionate debate over the impact of presumably disturbing or destructive target groups on society, but moreover because important policy options in all cases include a restriction of human rights. They seek to either remove target group members from the community by placing them into asylums, ghettos, work camps, prisons, or similar segregated environments, to deport them from the nation altogether, to remove their freedom to assemble, speak, or procreate, or, in the case of Nazi programs against the Jews and persons with cognitive or mental disabilities, to kill them outright. In such cases, the employment of dehumanizing or threat-inducing rhetoric is particularly necessary, since such actions run counter to important cultural beliefs, such as the acceptance of diversity, equal treatment, constitutionally based freedoms, and the right to due process.

Relevant metaphor themes

The five metaphor themes that are subject to description and analysis in this book include the following: (a) the organism metaphor, (b) the animal or subhuman metaphor, (c) the war and natural catastrophe metaphors, (d) the religious and altruistic metaphors, and (e) the object metaphor. Since they are described at length in the various chapters, I will only briefly introduce them here. Each of these themes may be employed either to dehumanize the group in question or to describe them as an imminent threat to society against which we must defend ourselves. There is a great deal of overlap between the various themes, and certain statements or images could include references to multiple metaphors. Since the themes do overlap with each other somewhat, certain examples may be appropriately delegated to more than one theme.

The organism metaphor is a means of describing the collective social body or nation as similar to a human body. The health of the whole requires that all elements of the organism work together toward common goals and to nurture the body. Importantly, like germs, bacteria, or viruses, target groups are often viewed as invasive or destructive social elements that are capable of infecting the mass of the community. Methods of control such as segregation, therefore, are often presented as community protection measures, similar to other forms of public health.

Through the animal metaphor, animalistic terminology or descriptions are used to highlight negative stereotyped characteristics of target group members. As Zuckier noted, propagandists may question where the boundary line that demarcates humans from non-human animals may be located, and whether target groups fall within or outside this line. The term 'marginalized' itself relates to this perception that group members should not be considered 'full-fledged' members of the human community.[37] Social movements often include elements of a 'scale of humanity' where various gradations of humans can be gauged, on the basis of racial, personal, behavioral, or other traits. Thus, even if all members of the species are accepted as human beings, some may be denied certain rights or opportunities on the basis of their placement on such a scale.

The war metaphor includes the extensive employment of military rhetoric or a general framing of the group in question as an imminent threat to the nation, whose control is warranted by the need to protect the community. While measures of control or restriction are generally undesirable, propagandists note, at times they are necessary because of the extreme nature of the threat. The war metaphor is also a means of highlighting the contention that, while there are many problems and issues facing the country, this particular concern is preeminent and must be faced immediately and forcefully. Like the war metaphor, the natural catastrophe metaphor portrays the group in question as analogous to a potentially cataclysmic act of nature.

The religious metaphor infuses religious rhetoric or symbolism within arguments for social control. The group in question is often portrayed as evil, immoral, or detrimental to the spiritual foundations of the community. Those supporting the movement will often take pains to demonstrate that its goals or methods are in keeping with mainstream religious precepts, and may even attempt to co-opt existing religious networks to disseminate propaganda. Similar is the altruistic metaphor, wherein social control is framed as a moral imperative directing those in power to control the group as a means of protecting or aiding the victims themselves.

Through the object metaphor, impersonal objects are used to highlight presumed characteristics of the target group. The value of group members is not a given, but may be based on their ability to perform specific roles, such as those of breeder, worker, soldier, and so on. They may be viewed as interchangeable objects with little individual personality, and the target classification – moron, Communist sympathizer, Japanese, Jew, and so on – may be presented by those in power as their 'master status' or principal identifying attribute. These primary identifiers, moreover, are often said to be largely unalterable.

Each of these five metaphor themes played a crucial role in support of eugenic arguments for controlling the procreative capacity of persons who were diagnosed as morons, as well as other undesirable subgroups of the population. The themes furthermore allowed eugenicists to present the case for eugenic reforms in a manner that could be easily understood by the general population. At the beginning of the twentieth century the term 'moron' did not exist, and therefore had no meaning. Within a few decades, morons were everywhere. They were weeds in our garden, cancers on our collective body, rapidly reproducing rats and viruses, weights on our shoulders, and a host of other pejorative images. We might conceptualize words as being vessels which carry meaning between persons. The following chapters demonstrate how the empty 'moron' vessel came to be filled by eugenic writers during the first quarter of the century.

Notes

1 Sections of this chapter were originally published in the author's 'Metaphors and the pejorative framing of marginalized groups: Implications for social work education', *Journal of Social Work Education* 45 (2009), 29–46.

2 B. Blatt, *Exodus from Pandomonium* (Boston: Allyn and Bacon, Inc., 1970), p. 161.

3 S.J. Gould, *Dinosaur in a Haystack* (New York: Harmony Books, 1995), pp. 443–4.

4 D.A. Schön, 'Generative metaphor: A perspective on problem-setting in social policy', in A. Ortony (ed.), *Metaphor and Thought* (New York: Cambridge University Press, 1979), p. 254.

5 See, for example, F. Krohn, 'Military metaphors', *Et Cetera: A Review of General Semantics* 44 (1987), 142; A. Harrington, 'Metaphoric connections: Holistic science in the shadow of the Third Reich', *Social Research* 62 (1995), 359; and W.N. Ellwood, 'Declaring war on the home front: Metaphor, presidents, and the war on drugs', *Metaphor and Symbolic Activity* 10:2 (1995), 93.

6 S. Sontag, *Illness as Metaphor and AIDS and its Metaphors* (New York: Anchor Books, 1990), p. 93.

7 Gould, *Dinosaur in a Haystack*, p. 444.

8 D.W. Allbritton, 'When metaphors function as schemas: Some cognitive effects of conceptual metaphors', *Metaphor and Symbolic Activity* 10 (1995), 36.

9 G. Lakoff, 'Metaphor, morality, and politics, or, Why conservatives have left liberals in the dust', *Social Research* 62 (1995), 177.

10 Schön, 'Generative metaphor', p. 265.

11 Allbritton, 'When metaphors function as schemas', p. 37; see also, Lakoff, 'Metaphor, morality, and politics', p. 182.

12 Allbritton, 'When metaphors function as schemas', p. 38.

13 G.A. De Vos and M.M. Suárez-Orozco, 'Sacrifice and the experience of power', in G.A. De Vos and M.M. Suárez-Orozco (eds.), *Status Inequality: The Self in Culture* (Newbury Park, CA: Sage Publications, 1990), p. 131.

14 W. Wolfensberger, *The Principle of Normalization in Human Services* (Toronto: National Institute on Mental Retardation, 1972), p. 16.

15 S. Keen, *Faces of the Enemy: Reflections of the Hostile Imagination* (San Francisco: Harper and Row, 1986), p. 13.

16 See N. Haslam, 'Dehumanization: An integrative review', *Personality and Social Psychology Review* 10 (2006), 252–64.

17 Schön, 'Generative metaphor', pp. 265–6.

18 B. Blatt, *The Conquest of Mental Retardation* (Austin, TX: Pro-Ed, 1987), p. 305.

19 W. Brennan, *Dehumanizing the Vulnerable: When Word Games Take Lives* (Chicago: Loyola University Press, 1995), p. 1.

20 Ibid., p. 3.

21 Ibid., p. 12.

22 H. Zuckier, 'The essential "other" and the Jew: From antisemitism to genocide', *Social Research* 63 (1996), 1117.

23 L. Noël, *Intolerance: A General Survey*, trans. A. Bennett (Montreal and Kingston: McGill-Queen's University Press, 1994), p. 79.

24 See, for example, M. Foucault, *Madness and Civilization*, trans. R. Howard (New York: Vintage Books, 1965); E. Goffman, *Asylums: Essays on the Social Situation of Mental Patients and Other Inmates* (Garden City, NY: Anchor Books, 1961),

and *Stigma* (Englewood Cliffs, NJ: Prentice-Hall, Inc., 1963); T. Szasz, *The Manufacture of Madness: A Comparative Study of the Inquisition and the Mental Health Movement* (New York: Harper and Row, 1970).

25 See, for example, T. Shakespeare, 'Cultural representation for disabled people: Dustbins for disavowal?', *Disability & Society* 9 (1994), 283–99; J.C. Drimmer, 'Cripples, overcomers, and civil rights: Tracing the evolution of federal legislation and social policy for people with disabilities', *UCLA Law Review* 40 (1993), 1341–410; and K. Fries (ed.), *Staring Back: The Disability Experience from the Inside Out* (New York: Penguin Putman, Inc., 1997).

26 Zuckier, 'The essential "other" and the Jew', p. 1118.

27 Noël, *Intolerance*, p. 7. Also see Paulo Freire's *Pedagogy of the Oppressed*, trans. M.B. Ramos, reprint edn. (New York: Continuum, 1986).

28 Allbritton, 'When metaphors function as schemas', p. 35. For specific examples of metaphor usage by politicians within the context of specific policy debates, see Elwood, 'Declaring war on the home front', and J.F. Voss, J. Kennet, J. Wiley, and T.Y.E. Schooler, 'Experts at debate: The use of metaphor in the U.S. Senate debate on the Gulf Crisis', *Metaphor and Symbolic Activity* 7 (1992), 197–214. For a more thorough discussion of the role of metaphor in social policy, see Lakoff's 'Metaphor, morality, and politics', or his more expansive *Moral Politics: What Conservatives Know that Liberals Don't* (Chicago and London: University of Chicago Press, 1996).

29 Lakoff, 'Metaphor, morality, and politics', p. 177.

30 Schön, 'Generative metaphor', p. 255.

31 Ibid., p. 266.

32 The term 'welfare' is extremely vague, but included because of its widespread use in popular nomenclature. In the United States there is no policy formally titled 'welfare'. The term has a range of meanings, but primarily has come to describe those receiving various forms of public assistance.

33 G.J. Annas, 'Reframing the debate on health care reform by replacing our metaphors', *New England Journal of Medicine* 332 (1995), 744–7.

34 Lakoff, *Moral Politics*.

35 Ellwood, 'Declaring war on the home front', p. 95. Also see, for example, M. Douglas's *Purity and Danger: An Analysis of the Concepts of Pollution and Taboo* (London: Routledge and Kegan Paul, 1966), and W.I. Miller's *The Anatomy of Disgust* (Cambridge, MA: Harvard University Press, 1997).

36 M.B. Levin, *Political Hysteria in America* (New York: Basic Books, Inc., 1971), p. 144.

37 Zuckier, 'The essential "other" and the Jew', p. 1123.

2

THE ORGANISM METAPHOR:
THE MORON AS A DISEASED ENTITY[1]

[C]rime and dependency keep on increasing because new defectives are born, just as new cancer cells remorselessly penetrate into sound tissues ... [i]t would by no means be a misnomer to call the American Eugenics Society a Society for the Control of Social Cancer.[2]

Ostracized community groups are often portrayed as diseased entities that threaten to infect, contaminate, and corrupt the healthy components of the social body. Linguistic metaphors that are a central feature of the larger organism metaphor, such as those of plague, cancer, and virus, are increasingly prevalent within contemporary sociopolitical dialogue. It seems to be almost a daily occurrence that a new group of social outcasts or a different social problem is described as a plague upon society or a source of societal contamination from which we must protect ourselves and our children. While this disease rhetoric is the primary defining characteristic of the organism metaphor, other pejorative modes of describing the presumed adverse impact of the target group on society also come into play. These will be described below.

The University of Chicago sociologist Donald Levine described the historical significance of the organism metaphor, noting that comparisons between human and national or community bodies extend back thousands of years.[3] Through this metaphor the community or a nation is depicted as a biological entity, similar in many ways to the human body. What are perceived to be homogenous groups of people are conceptualized as constituent components of this organic body. The value of these collectives presumably depends on the extent to which they can be viewed as contributing to overall societal functioning. As Levine noted, '[p]erhaps the greatest range of uses to which the organism metaphor has been put appears in its service as a vehicle for normative judgments about social conditions'.[4] In his book *Metaphor and Political Discourse*, Andreas Musolff describes the organism metaphor in detail, noting that the metaphor 'has had a long tradition in political discourse and thought, dating back to antiquity and permutating over the centuries'.[5] Musolff provides a wealth of examples of the recent use of the metaphor in contemporary European political speeches.

It is useful to consider the organism metaphor chronologically, following its progress from efforts to identify the potentially dangerous entities, to the feared penetration, contamination, and spread of the entities within the social body, and ending with the eventual disease, death, and decay of the previous healthy organism because of inadequate methods of prevention. The only way to protect the healthy social body is to isolate the unhealthy, disease-carrying elements, or to ensure they do not penetrate community or national boundaries.[6] Thus policies related to institutionalization, community or national gatekeeping, imprisonment, deportation, or even elimination of the unhealthy organisms are the forms of social control that most clearly relate to the organism metaphor.

As noted above, a prevalent theme in the use of the organism metaphor is the contamination of the healthy segments of society by the unhealthy components. Metaphors related to contagion may be viewed as an extreme form of animalization. Conceptually, the animal metaphor grades over into the organism metaphor as the animals become ever smaller and more inconsequential, becoming, in the end, germs, viruses, and cancer cells. Those groups that can be perceived as invasive and destructive tumors or parasites within society can be acted on with relative impunity. Intolerance, Lise Noël said, 'takes on an almost immunological form, with the healthy antibodies of society violently rejecting what it perceives as "foreign" elements'.[7]

Perhaps the most important advocate of this perceptual image was Herbert Spencer, the foremost advocate of social Darwinism.[8] Spencer wrote in 1904 that 'a society as a whole, considered apart from its living units, presents phenomena of growth, structure, and function, like those of growth, structure, and function in an individual body'. He added that a 'metaphor, when used to express a real resemblance, raises a suspicion of mere imaginary resemblance; and so obscures the perception of intrinsic kinship'.[9] As Levine noted, Spencer believed that the state was a living organism, not just symbolically, but in a very real sense.[10]

George Chatterton-Hill, in his 1907 book *Heredity and Selection in Sociology*, expanded on this application of the organism metaphor. An Irish writer, Chatterton-Hill was a follower of Spencer, and he not only equated society to a physical body but also compared the individuals making up that society to the food taken in by a biological organism. Some food, he said, representing the more fit or desirable segments of society, serves to provide essential nutrients. This food is incorporated within the social body and assists in energizing it and ensuring its survival. Other types of food, presumably having a similar effect on the body to unfit and diseased societal elements, are depicted as little more than waste products. They cannot serve the body, and the inability of the organism to properly eliminate this food – or to effectively guard against ingesting it in the first place – could even be detrimental to the organism, and potentially lethal.[11] Henry Fairchild, one of the foremost supporters of immigration restriction in the United States, described the assimilation of immigrant groups by comparing the immigrant to the food that is taken in by a body. Discussing this analogy, he contended that 'there is such a close resemblance between a human society and a living organism that the analogy if not abused may serve a distinct purpose in clarifying the concepts involved'.[12]

The fear of the target group as a symbolic virus or source of contamination is often heightened when its members are presented as insidiously 'hiding' within the 'general population'. Like Mary Mallon (Typhoid Mary), the Irish immigrant who had no symptoms of typhoid but spread the disease to a number of others, they may not present with any symptoms of the disease that they can pass on to others. In such cases, the scope of social control may be expanded to include all persons within the group who are potentially threatening. In the most extreme cases, such as Japanese internment, the difficulty of differentiating the harmful from the non-threatening members of the group may be said to necessitate that social control measures be taken against virtually all those who belong to the group, even when very few are found to be actually engaging in harmful activities.

Additionally, as an outgrowth of this inability to distinguish easily which members of the group should be subject to social measures, a cadre of 'diagnosticians', 'investigators', or law-enforcement professionals who can presumably separate the threatening members of the group from the rest of the community will be created. The rise in diagnostic or investigatory expertise naturally leads to a rapid increase in the number of persons who fall within the target class, thus resulting in an exacerbation in the fear that such persons are indeed penetrating and contaminating the community. This increase in numbers and the presumption of threat reinforces the need for and expansion of the 'investigatory infrastructure'. As in the case of the eugenics movement, this cycle often continues until it implodes under its own weight.

The spread of an infected sub-population within society is frequently presented as a form of cancer or a rapidly growing virus. Such spread is often said to occur through the presumptive high fecundity of group members, or by their intermarriage or sexual relations with persons outside the group. As with the Jews in Nazi Germany or African-Americans in the segregated South of the United States, the target group may be depicted as 'poisoning' the blood of the nation. One Nazi leader, for example, argued that the semen of male Jews was so corrupting that once a Jew had had sexual relations with an Aryan women, she could never again have an 'untainted' child, even if the child was the product of a later union with a fellow Aryan.[13] Spread may also occur through covert recruitment of members or through the group's perceived control of the media or important governmental institutions, leading to the spread of its ideology or value system, or other methods of disseminating 'destructive' information or values.

Propagandists argue that the only way to protect the nation that is threatened by potentially infectious subgroups is to keep them out of the 'general population', to quarantine them until it is certain they pose no further threat, or to perform a radical 'surgical' intervention to exterminate the infectious portion of the social body. Spencer discussed this surgical analogy in his book *Social Statics*:

> We should think it a very foolish sort of benevolence which led a surgeon to let his patient's disease progress to a fatal issue, rather than inflict pain by an operation. Similarly, we must call those spurious philanthropists who, to prevent present misery, would entail greater misery on future generations ... Blind to the fact that under the natural order of things society is constantly excreting its unhealthy, imbecile, slow, vacillating, faithless members, these unthinking, though well-meaning, men advocate an interference which not only stops the purifying process, but even increases the vitiation.[14]

When the 'disease' has gained a foothold in society and quarantine is no longer an option, extermination of the 'infected' components of the population may be presented as the only way of ensuring the survival of the community. Certainly the clearest examples of this application of the organism metaphor were Nazi Germany's race hygiene programs. A number of scholars have noted that, in keeping with the Nazis' focus on race purity, Nazi medicine was much more concerned with the health of the social body than with the physical well-being of individuals.[15] Within this context, the physician, or 'genetic doctor', was a healer not of individuals, but of the state, and, just as an inflamed appendix would be removed from a diseased body, a diseased individual was viewed as inimical to the future health of the *Volk*.[16]

The organism metaphor and the menace of the feeble-minded

The last quarter of the nineteenth century and first quarter of the twentieth were characterized in part by the expanding influence of a medically based conceptualization of the world. The growth in medical science naturally led to efforts to employ this knowledge to provide both an explanation of and treat-ments for large-scale social problems. In keeping with a scientific mindset that gave credence to nature over nurture (especially following the rediscovery of Mendel's laws in 1900), Robert Ward wrote in the midst of the eugenic era that 'it is becoming clear that the day of the sociologist is passing, and the day of the biologist has come',[17] and Lothrop Stoddard stated that biology was the 'champion of the new'.[18] The Harvard professor Earnest Hooton added that 'a biological purge is the essential prerequisite for a social and spiritual salvation' within the country, and society 'must stop trying to cure malignant biological growths with patent sociological nostrums'. 'The emergency', he concluded, speaking of the procreation of the unfit, 'demands a surgical operation.'[19]

The ascension of medical science in the early part of the twentieth century, especially genetics and public health, played an important role in the wide-spread employment of the organism metaphor within the context of the eugen-ics movement. Those who were classified as feeble-minded were frequently described in the writings of eugenicists as diseased organisms, reproducing at an alarming rate and infecting the 'healthy' portions of the community. They were said to be a 'an ulcer on our social tissue',[20] 'a festering ulcer on our country's breast',[21] and 'an insidious disease affecting the body politic'.[22] Leon Stern, talking about the 'Bilder clan', a family on which he conducted eugenic research, said that to 'dig into the records of their social life is to dig into an ulcer in the community that is spread and ramified'.[23] In the same vein, Martin Barr, a leading institutional administrator from Pennsylvania, wrote that '[w]herever defect or disease rests unguarded, it becomes a festering sore, sure to eat as a canker or in some sudden unexpected outbreak to cause ruin to many'.[24]

Primarily, however, such individuals were compared to a cancer or tumor. Florence Sherbon, a leader in the movement to bring eugenics to main-stream America through the 'Fitter Families' contests, wrote that 'unrestrained propagation of the unfit presents a phenomenon not unlike the wild cells of a malignant growth which devour and destroy their host and thus, eventu-ally, themselves'.[25] In his book *Tomorrow's Children* Ellsworth Huntington included a rather extensive section comparing eugenics to cancer treatment.[26] In describing the reproduction rate of morons, another eugenicist stated that while '[a] few segregated and magnified germs are interesting objects of agree-able study ... a colony of the same germs become a horrifying mass of cancer-ous corruption'.[27]

As these quotations illustrate, cancer was specifically used to highlight the differential fecundity argument, as morons were perceived to be multiply-ing quickly and imperceptibly, like the cells of a malignant tumor. Lothrop

Stoddard believed that feeble-minded individuals were 'spreading like cancerous growths, disturbing the social life and infecting the blood of whole communities' and 'threatening to corrode society to the very marrow of its being'.[28] The subjects of the eugenic family studies were described in a 1938 *Reader's Digest* article as 'human cancers in our social organism'.[29] Regarding concerns that large-scale eugenic programs might wrongly diagnose some 'normal' persons, leading to their sterilization or institutionalization, Sherbon contended that '[t]he surgeon removes much normal tissue with the cancerous growth but feels justified in that he knows no other way of saving the organism itself'. She expressed the hope that at some future date a safer and more accurate method of treating both cancer and social degeneracy would be discovered. Until this occurred, however, 'the radical operation' was the only option for both.[30]

Pollution and the spread of moronity

In some eugenic writings, the rapid spread of feeble-mindedness was described in terms where the analogy to clinical cytology is unmistakable. Discussing the 'Ishmaels', a family that was the subject of an Indiana eugenic study, Albert Wiggam wrote:

> A few generations ago there were but two of them [Ishmaels] to care for, only two of them to suffer from disease, feeble-mindedness, filth, and incompetence, only two of them to spread crime, pauperism, prostitution, and disease throughout the community; but as a result of this policy of caring for them and *doing nothing else*, there are now nearly twelve thousand![31]

Many eugenicists contended that there was little substantive difference between the impurities and diseases that threatened the human body and the feeble-minded subgroup, which was the primary source of 'pollution' that endangered the social body. Preventive mechanisms as a means of protection, moreover, were just as important in each case.[32] Charles Davenport, the leading American eugenicist, asked readers, in response to the eugenic family studies, whether they would rouse themselves if they learned 'there were ten cases of bubonic plague at a point not 200 miles away.' He then asked whether 'a breeding pot of uncontrolled animalism is as much of a menace to our civilization'.[33] He also wrote that while a new plague would arouse the attention of the nation and attract a great deal of money for research and prevention, 'we have become so used to crime, disease and degeneracy that we take them as necessary evils'.[34] Decrying the fact that society did not have an organized plan for sterilizing or institutionalizing morons, Martin Barr said that 'it does seem absurd that while we wage war upon microbes and bacilli, we turn loose this worse than leprosy to poison the very springs of life'.[35] Several years later he added that '[w]e guard against all epidemics, are quick to quarantine small-pox, and we exclude the Chinese; but take no steps to eliminate this evil from the social body'.[36] A 1912 letter to the editor published in the *Survey*, an important social reform journal of the time, held that '[i]t is just as possible to prevent the birth of delinquents, idiots, feeble-minded, hereditary criminals, and hereditary paupers as it is to prevent typhoid and yellow fever; why isn't it done?'[37]

Morons were perceived to be a greater source of contamination than imbeciles and idiots, not only because they procreated more, but also since they graded into the 'regular' population. As described above, when target group members cannot be readily identified they tend to solicit more fear, just as an asymptomatic carrier of disease invites panic since he or she may be anyone with whom we come into contact. Eugenicists played on this theme, noting, for example, that the evil represented by the moron was 'all the more dangerous because it is insidious'.[38] The author of the Kallikak study, Henry Goddard, ominously warned his readers that there were 'Kallikak families all about us'.[39] That the average individual could not tell the moron from the 'normal' person was all the more reason, moreover, to provide authority for those who contended that they could, such as intelligence testers and institutional administrators. As diagnostic expertise expanded, the perceived community of morons quickly increased to an extraordinary degree.

As a malignancy or plague within society, feeble-minded individuals were viewed as an actual or feared source of contamination, pollution, and infection.[40] They threatened to transmit their malignancy throughout the rest of the community, largely by means of intermarriage or intercourse with persons who were not feeble-minded. 'Normal strains', a eugenicist noted, were 'becoming contaminated with anti-social and defective traits.'[41] Another referred to a feeble-minded child as a 'new stream of contamination' within society.[42] When supporters of eugenics lobbied in state legislatures for sterilization laws or increased institutional funding, they often displayed charts from the family studies. These presentations showed, in graphic detail, 'the vitiating spread of mental defectiveness throughout a whole stock'.[43] Discussing the prevailing view of the 'immigrating underclass', many of whom were taken to be morons, Betsy Nies concluded that 'the nation itself became figured as a body that would sicken and die if infested with such carriers of social disorders'.[44]

A clear example of how the organism metaphor served as an apt means of framing the need for eugenic control is included below. Here Joseph Byers, the Commissioner of the New Jersey Commission of Charities and Correction, refers to Elizabeth Kite's study, under the direction of Henry Goddard, of the 'Piney' families, a large New Jersey family assumed to be composed mostly of individuals of poor stock:

> The objects of the investigation ... were, first, 'to know the sources of the con-
> tamination that is polluting the stream of our social life'; second, 'to cleanse or
> cut off the sources of pollution'; third, 'to quarantine until cured all who have
> been infected'. This is an allegorical way of putting the problem, but the parallel
> between the prevention of breeding of anti-social stock and the location and
> stamping out of disease at its source, is so close that the analogy is a good one.[45]

Many eugenicists contended that the virulence of 'bad' blood was such that it would overwhelm and destroy 'good' blood. According to Henry Goddard, author of the Kallikak study, 'cacogenic' or defective descendants of Martin Kallikak[46] appeared to have few if any of his characteristics after his blood had been 'contaminated by that of the nameless feeble-minded girl'.[47] The Wisconsin zoology professor and eugenicist Michael Guyer added that when others mated with members of the Kallikak family, instead of their 'redeeming the tainted stock', the 'new blood ... itself became vitiated'.[48] In another work this author wrote that 'we cannot continue to drink the sluggish blood of the pauper and the imbecile into our veins and hope to escape unscathed'.[49] Drawing on an early, simplistic form of Mendelism, many eugenicists perceived the human species to be composed of 'pure' and 'impure' strains, and that the primary goal of eugenics was to ensure that 'the family lines of pure strain shall not be contaminated'.[50]

Some not only used contagious disease metaphors to describe the potential impact of defectives on the community, but literally contended that effectively dealing with feeble-mindedness through eugenic measures would largely diminish the spread of transmissible diseases within the country. As morons were viewed as the seminal source of many other social problems, they were also said to be primarily responsible for the proliferation of venereal diseases. Helen MacMurchy, a Canadian physician who specialized in feeble-mindedness, spoke on this relationship before the 1916 National Conference on Charities and Correction. 'Do you', she asked, 'seek a focus of contagious disease? Are you wondering where the "carriers" are? Have you a register of the feeble-minded of the city in the office of the medical officer of health? You will seldom miss your mark if you begin there.'[51]

Morons, especially the females, were considered to be the primary purveyors of venereal diseases because of their presumed lax morality and diminished control over their carnal urges. 'One perverted feeble-minded woman', Amos Butler wrote in 1901, 'can spread throughout a community an immoral pestilence which will affect the homes of all classes, even the most intelligent and refined.'[52] Statements such as the following one, written by Walter Fernald, who operated the major institution for feeble-minded persons in Massachusetts, are found throughout eugenic writings, and present the image of female morons as a wellspring of contagion;

> It is well known that feeble-minded women and girls are very liable to become sources of unspeakable debauchery and licentiousness which pollutes the whole life of the young boys and youth of the community. They frequently disseminate in a wholesale way the most loathsome and deadly diseases, permanently poisoning the minds and bodies of thoughtless youth at the very threshold of manhood.[53]

While some eugenicists portrayed feeble-minded women as ignorant victims of exploitative males, others depicted them as being evil seductresses knowingly contaminating unsuspecting men. Whatever their complicity in spreading their taint, however, the recommendations put forth by eugenicists did not vary. Eugenic measures alone would protect society from such women. For those who saw them as innocent perpetrators of immorality, moreover, institutionalization was altruistically viewed as a measure that would protect them from those males who would take advantage of them if they were left 'unguarded' in the community. Elizabeth Yukins, in her analysis of the portrayal of females in eugenic family studies, describes at some length the extent to which women such as Deborah Kallikak 'were pathologized as dangerous biological contaminants'. Within the context of these studies, she noted, the utilization of biological metaphors primarily related to the sexual behavior of lower-class women.[54] As noted in the Introduction, it was far from coincidental that the era within which the eugenics movement thrived in the United States was a period when many women were seeking (and, in many cases, attaining) new freedoms, including increased reproductive knowledge and sexual autonomy. Those women who were diagnosed as or even simply perceived to be 'morons' may have served as convenient scapegoats for those who felt threatened or discomforted by such expanding freedoms.

Filth, contagion, and the moron

The perception of the target group as dirty, filthy, or unhygienic is often a precursor to viewing its members as a diseased entity. It also serves to reinforce the animalistic metaphor that such persons are subhuman beings. Since filth causes disease, those social groups that live in unsanitary conditions are especially likely to carry and spread communicable diseases. Indeed, their predilection to filth may be said to imbue them with a tolerance or immunity to the diseases they carry. In addition to their propensity to spread venereal disease, the filthy environments within which many of the poor feeble-minded were said to live presumably subjected them to the full range of transmissible diseases. 'Have you ever, anywhere, and under any circumstances', MacMurchy wrote, 'smelt anything to compare with the indescribable, compressed, complex, horrible odor of the air in one of these abodes of the feeble-minded?'[55] A central feature of the eugenic family studies was the graphic depictions of the subhuman, primitivistic environs of 'rural morons'. These studies were replete with photographs and descriptions of broken-down shanties, unsanitary conditions, and children who lacked even the most basic hygiene.[56] One such home that Elizabeth Kite visited as part of the Kallikak study was described as follows:

> The hideous picture that presented itself as the door opened to her [the field worker's] knock was one never to be forgotten ... In one arm she [the 'imbecile' mother] held a frightful looking baby, while she had another by the hand. Vermin were visible all over her. In the room were a few chairs and a bed, the latter without any washable covering and filthy beyond description ... The oldest girl, a vulgar, repulsive creature of fifteen, came into the room and stood looking at the stranger. She had somehow managed to live.[57]

As Nicole Hahn Rafter pointed out in *White Trash*, her seminal book on the family studies, such images abound in these works.[58] As noted above, it was in this pervasive image of the feeble-minded person as a filthy, vermin-ridden subhuman that the organism metaphor merged with the animal metaphor. Lice, parasites, and other such entities are both animals and sources of contagion. They therefore are an apt metaphor for the highly fecund but undesirable social group, not only animalizing them, but additionally characterizing members as a threat to the health of the social body. The parasitic nature of mental defectives, noted Eugene Talbot, was an important indicator of its atavistic or primitive state.[59] The famous social critic and writer H.L. Mencken, in justifying a proposed sterilization program for the rural poor, many of whom he presumed to be feeble-minded, wrote that:

> The birth rate, down in those pious and malarious wastes ... is precisely what the traffic will bear, and if it were not for the fact that the death rate, especially among children, is also inordinate, the region would swarm like a nest of maggots.[60]

There can also be little doubt that the conditions in which the subjects of the family studies lived contributed greatly to a diagnosis of feeble-mindedness. The rater's predisposition against a 'lower-class' environment no doubt could lead her to classify individuals who lived within these surroundings more harshly than otherwise would have been the case. To Kite and many of the other authors of family studies, who came largely from middle- and upper-class families, there is little doubt that the depravity of lower-class environs was in itself fairly indicative of moronity.[61] 'Like other eugenicists', Rafter wrote, these authors 'were not just promoting a new set of public policies but engaged in an almost religious crusade for class preservation and aggrandizement'.[62]

A core feature of this middle-class mentality was the Protestant work ethic, and a continuing theme in eugenic writings was the laziness and dependency of the moron. Feeble-minded persons, eugenicists wrote, were parasitic entities that took from the community without giving anything back. They were described as 'barnacles upon our civilization',[63] 'a parasitic class',[64] which was allowed to 'breed like lice',[65] and a 'fungus growth' that was 'fastening itself upon the unfortunate community'.[66] Perhaps one of the most interesting parasitic equivalents proposed for the dysgenic person was the Sacculina, described by Oscar McCulloch in the early study of the family he called the 'Ishmaels'. According to Nathaniel Deutsch, who described the study in a 2009 book, the Sacculina was a small crustacean that 'attached to the body of its host, the hermit crab'. As with other parasites (including human ones, McCulloch hypothesized), a hereditary defect had led the animal to become dependent on another entity, and had led to its degeneration over time, as it had evolved to the point where it was no longer capable of independently meeting its important needs.[67]

Caroline Robinson described the effect that 'degenerate' elements of the population had on tax-payers by saying that that the latter were 'already supporting one public parasite per solvent family'.[68] The feeble-minded were not just a benign parasite that could exist side by side with their host with no harm being done. Rather, Leon Cole wrote, they were 'sapping at the vigor, the health, the happiness, the social morality, and the civic cleanliness of the nation'.[69] Eugenic measures, wrote Sherbon, would ensure that the 'unfit' could be preserved but would 'not retaliate by devouring their host', which was the community within which they lived.[70]

A public health response to the problem

As the moron class came to be depicted as a public health catastrophe, fostered in large part by misguided philanthropy, only a public health solution, eugenicists argued, could save the nation from corruption and eventual decomposition. Earnest Hooton said that humankind was like Noah's Ark, and that if we were to survive we must 'leave out some of the noxious animals who are boring from within and making that ark dangerously leaky'. 'It behooves us', he continued, 'to learn our human parasitology and human entomology, to practise an artificial and scientific selection with intelligence, if we wish to save our skins.'[71] To the eugenicists, Martin Pernick wrote, '[h]ereditary diseases were as threatening as contagious epidemics'. He quoted Dr Haiselden, who championed the infanticide of disabled newborns, as comparing 'eugenic sterilization to "shoot[ing] down a slobbering cur in the streets to prevent it from spreading its rabies"'. 'The unfit', Pernick continued in The Black Stork, 'did not simply *have* a disease, they *were* the disease.'[72]

Some advocates of long-term institutionalization referred to segregation as a public health measure. Since 'the degeneracy of the feeble-minded is transmissible', the superintendent of the New Jersey facility argued, only long-term placement would save society from the 'grave dangers' posed by such persons.[73] Following the Kallikak study, the Governor of New Jersey recommended segregating the Pine Barrens, where most of the family was thought to reside, from the rest of the state for public health purposes.[74] Isolating the 'carriers of mental defect', said one writer, was more important than other forms of quarantine, since the 'sum of human misery in this country due to every contagious disease is not one-tenth that entailed by mental defect'.[75] Some referred to segregation as 'sexual quarantine',[76] and others suggested that institutions be located in remote areas, as if the placement of such facilities in urban areas created a risk to the surrounding population even if the residents were kept in a segregated state.[77] Martin Barr, for example, recommended that a national institution be developed on an isolated island,[78] while Charles Bernstein, a fellow institutional administrator, noted but was critical of the suggestion that 'an institution for women of child-bearing age [be] located on waste land in a territory removed far from civilization'.[79]

Sterilization too was touted as a public health measure when invoked for eugenic purposes. As Pernick wrote, a close conceptual relationship existed between germs and 'germ plasm', which meant genes during the better part of the eugenic era. Both enabled 'diseases to propagate, spreading lethal contamination from guilty to innocent bodies', and both could be effectively eradicated by means of sterilization.[80] In its 1927 Buck v. Bell decision, the United States Supreme Court acknowledged the societal benefits of involuntary sterilization by comparing the procedure to compulsory vaccination.[81] Citing the earlier Jacobson v. Massachusetts case, the court held that 'the police power of the State must be held to embrace, at least, such reasonable regulations established directly by legislative enactment as will protect the public health and the public safety'.[82] E.S. Gosney, the President of the Human Betterment Foundation and leader of California's sterilization campaign, quoted a Viennese surgeon who supported sterilization because it was 'the duty of medicine to prevent disease and this is one means of prevention'.[83] Clarence Gamble, a physician and supporter of eugenics, wrote of hereditary diseases that since 'the "incubation period" of these "diseases" covers so many years before they are recognized, physicians and laymen are apt to forget that they are contagious and that tubectomy [tubal ligation] can provide the "isolation" which contagious diseases require'. He went on to write that '[v]isualization of feebleminded children who are not born requires as much mental effort as the imagining of the smallpox epidemics which vaccination keeps from occurring'.[84] Heritability, many eugenicists argued, was really no different from any other form of disease transmission, and needed to be treated as such.

Supporters also invoked the organism metaphor in arguing that restrictive immigration laws would also serve to protect the nation from the large mass of feeble-minded and defective immigrants who were 'supplanting good stocks'. As Lothrop Stoddard wrote:

> Just as we isolate bacterial invasions, and starve out the bacteria by limiting the area and amount of their food-supply, so we can compel an inferior race to remain in its native habitat, where its own multiplication in a limited area will, as with all organisms, eventually limit its numbers and therefore its influence.[85]

Immigration restrictionists frequently referred to those coming into the country, especially from eastern and southern Europe, as 'indigestible' food that could not be absorbed in such large quantities by the national body, or even as poisonous elements.[86] Employing an 'immigrant as food' metaphor that is frequently found in such writings, one questioned whether the push to force limitations on immigration was due only to the fact that 'the food is strange and alien, or does it possibly contain poisons against which we have no antidote?'[87] Keeping the 'diseased' elements of a target group out of the general population was presented by others as little different from protecting the water supply and similar public health measures:

> The theoretically perfect control of immigration is much the same in principle as that exercised over community water supply. To see that it is plentiful, that it is of the best quality, free from possible pollution at the source, and that it is properly distributed, is the duty of a popular Government.[88]

Robert Ward, one of the leaders of the immigration restriction movement in the United States, decried the potential public health impact of the nation's inability to keep out potentially feeble-minded and otherwise undesirable immigrants. He noted that we should 'exercise the same care in admitting human beings as we exercise in relation to animals or insect pests or disease germs'.[89]

Just as persons with certain infectious diseases were required by the state to be registered, some advocates of eugenics recommended that those with feeble-mindedness and other degenerate conditions likewise be registered for public health purposes. Walter Fernald, for example, said that a precedent had been set for registration of the feeble-minded, since 'state commissions for controlling the gypsy moth and the boll weevil, [and] the foot-and-mouth disease' already existed,[90] and in another article he noted that 'registration would be merely analogous to the required notification and record of cases of infectious and contagious disease'.[91]

According to Pernick, Dr Haiselden, one of the few supporters of eugenics in the United States to openly advocate euthanasia as a eugenic measure, clearly invoked the organism metaphor by contending that the death of inferiors 'is the great and lasting disinfectant' for the nation.[92] While few mainstream American eugenicists publicly supported euthanasia as a eugenic response, many invoked eliminationist rhetoric that corresponded to the organism metaphor. 'Death', said Leon Cole, 'is the normal process of elimination in the social organism, and ... in prolonging the lives of defectives we are tampering with the functioning of the social kidneys.'[93] As in Nazi Germany, this rhetoric fostered the view that eliminating or preventing the birth of degenerates was an important element of purification or cleansing the community of its inferior elements. In 1929 Harry Laughlin of the Eugenics Record Office wrote an article for a German journal, wherein he stated that '[t]he racial hygienist as a biologist regards the development of eugenic sterilization as the effort of the state "organism" to get rid of the burden of its degenerate members'.[94] Lothrop Stoddard similarly stated, a full ten years before Hitler was elected chancellor, that the 'elimination of inferiors is a process of race cleansing' and that eugenic policies would 'cleanse the race of its worst impurities'.[95]

While the primary subject of this book is the eugenics movement in the United States, a brief mention of German eugenics under the Hitler regime is important here, especially as the Nazis' view of the world was strongly informed by the organism metaphor, and it particularly influenced their eugenic policies.[96] Among other writers, Paul Weindling has discussed the relationship between the organism metaphor and racial hygiene in Nazi Germany. He notes that the relationship between the state and the body was extensively exploited to support German policies against not only the Jews, but persons with disabilities and other disfavored groups. In fact, the term 'racial hygiene' itself demonstrates this connection.[97] He adds that '[t]he lethal trinity of showers, crematoria, and poison gas chambers had their origins in sanitary reform'.[98]

Hitler himself repeatedly employed the metaphor within the pages of *Mein Kampf*, frequently comparing Jews and other 'enemies of the state' to plagues, bacteria, tumors, parasites, lice, and other specters of disease.[99] Perhaps the most extensive description of Hitler's use of the organism metaphor was provided by Musolff in a 2007 article that appeared in the journal *Patterns of Prejudice*. Musolff deconstructs the use of metaphors throughout Hitler's manifesto, focusing primarily on the organism metaphor, and describes the historical underpinnings that supported Hitler's conception of the nation as a physical body. Within this perspective, eugenic measures, including elimination, were a proper means of dealing with potentially infectious entities or population subgroups.[100]

As noted above, Nazi medicine was directed at primarily serving what one might refer to as the 'body of the nation' over individual bodies. In other words, 'treatments' such as involuntary sterilization were seen as not only appropriate but a duty of physicians since they protected the spread of degeneracy throughout the nation.[101] The German government under Hitler viewed its eugenic programs as a necessary means of protecting society from genetic contagion from feeble-minded persons and other degenerate groups. Dr Guett, who wrote the 1933 sterilization law, noted that this policy was the 'most important public-health measure since the discovery of bacteria by another German enabled humanity to rid itself of plagues'.[102] Hitler himself is quoted as saying that the state needed to engage in eugenic policies in relation to feeble-minded and other degenerate persons since one of its duties was 'curing the national body of this sore'.[103]

In keeping with the organism metaphor as a means of framing its eugenic and race hygiene programs, the Nazis referred to gassing, first used in the T-4 euthanasia program, as *Desinfektion*,[104] and those who carried the bodies from the gas chambers to either the dissection rooms or incinerators were called 'disinfectors' or 'decontaminators'.[105] Zyklon B, used in the Auschwitz gas chambers, was originally developed by a fumigation company for the purpose of pest control.[106] Orders for the chemical 'were placed by the chief disinfectant officer of the Waffen SS on behalf of the Auschwitz "Extermination and Fumigation Division"',[107] and the gas was supplied by a company called Degesch, a name which was a German acronym for 'German Company for Pest Control'.[108]

Discussion

Since microscopic biology provided demonstrable proof of how undesirable cells could rapidly reproduce and overwhelm healthy organisms, it served as an apt means of representing the need for eugenic control. As will be further discussed in Chapter 7, the recurrent use of disease rhetoric in eugenic writings in both the United States and Nazi Germany was fostered in part by the biological orientation of the movement's leadership. Persons who tended to perceive problems from a biological framework might naturally extend this framework to their view of society in general. Additionally, interest in eugenics grew at a time when public health and medical innovation were important public concerns. Efforts to create community clinics, minimize occupationally related health hazards, control the spread of contagious diseases, ensure prompt garbage collection in urban areas, and foster clean food and water policies were among the many public health goals of the Progressive movement. While most components of the movement were 'euthenic' in nature, in that they were attempts to improve public health through environmental reforms, many believed that euthenics and eugenics needed to work together in order to achieve real progress. Environmental reforms without eugenic control would be viewed by many as similar to responding to a contagious disease simply by treating the symptoms and not the underlying source.

The organism metaphor was also an apt metaphor to employ in framing the moron population because of the close relationship that propagandists built between feeble-mindedness and the 'new' immigrants during the first decades of the century. This is especially true since the foreign origin of the target group is a central feature of the organism metaphor. Just as those elements that adversely affect the human body are usually seen as infecting us from the outside, so too those groups that contaminate the social body are frequently said to have a foreign origin. The target group, like a plague, is invariably viewed as coming from somewhere else. '[T]here is a link', Susan Sontag wrote, 'between imagining disease and imagining foreignness'.[109]

It should be noted that even when the social groups that are deemed to be harmful to the general population were born to standing members of the community, rationales that support a foreign identity may still be constructed. Such was the case, for example, with the Jews in Germany, who, regardless of their tenure within the country, still were said to embody a foreign nature or essence. Japanese-Americans too were considered, regardless of their families' tenure within the country, to be 'Japanese' and were therefore subject to internment. Likewise, feeble-minded persons, even if they were third- or fourth-generation Americans, were often characterized by eugenicists as the products of devalued foreign stock.

The organism metaphor was not only an important means of describing both the moron and the undesirable immigrant population. It also provided a conceptual basis for combining these two grave social problems, with each fear gaining strength as a result of this juxtaposition. The eugenic family studies and their descriptions of rapidly propagating parasitic feeble-minded families showed policymakers what supposedly happened to undesirable immigrants once they took up residence within the country. The immigrant, moreover, was the consummate outsider, the bearer of disease. It was in the specter of the moron or immigrant that the contaminating presence of the immigrant united with the genetic contaminant that was the moron. Moreover, both groups were presented as defilers of the race. 'Race suicide' became a pervasive fear during the early 1900s not only because 'native' American families were becoming smaller, but additionally because these other groups were supposedly increasing in size.

Reification of the metaphor

Interestingly, those subgroups that are subject to the organism metaphor as a primary means of social construction are often relegated to environments where they are apt to become infected with communicable diseases or parasites, thus reifying the metaphor. Ghettos, tenements, reservations, detention centers, immigrant work camps, prisons, asylums, and similar locations, as well as the vehicles used to transport people to such environments, are often characterized by unsanitary and unhealthy conditions. As contamination rates within such segregated facilities or settings increases, the perception that the group itself is infectious – and that its segregation is a public health concern rather than a social or political one – becomes validated. While Jews in Nazi Germany, for example, were referred to as 'lice' and 'bacteria' prior to their placement in ghettos and work camps, this metaphor was no doubt strengthened when they were placed in these environments, where they naturally acquired parasites and contagious diseases.[110]

Likewise, those who have been labeled feeble-minded or mentally retarded have historically been confined to institutional environments that have served to ensure that group members would indeed become a public health menace. This is not to imply that such placement occurs for the express purpose of reifying the metaphor. Nevertheless, the relationship between rhetoric that emphasizes images of contagion and contamination and the eventual infectious condition of group members cannot be lost on those who engage in or support social control measures.[111]

At times the infectious nature of some members of the target group is assured in an even more direct way than by placing them in contaminated environs. In Nazi Germany, not only Jews but the members of other undesirable classes were purposefully infected with disease agents for the purpose of researching the course of these diseases. More recently, in the United States a number of mentally retarded residents at the Willowbrook institution in

New York were purposefully infected with hepatitis from the late 1950s into the 1970s for the purpose of studying the course of the disease. Additionally, children at the Fernald School in Massachusetts were purposefully given cereal laced with radioactive isotopes during the 1940s and 1950s in order to study the long-term impact of radiation on the body. Especially in the case of the Willowbrook study, it seems to be true that the perception that these 'subjects' would eventually become contaminated anyway helped the researchers to justify the experiment.[112]

While it is now less extensive than in the past, the employment of the organism metaphor to describe the presumptive impact that persons with cognitive disabilities are said to have on society still plays an important role in framing such persons.[113] As concerns about the 'pollution' of the gene pool continue, especially in light of new genetic developments and increased opportunities to allow the prospective parents of a disabled child to abort, we will likely see an increase the organism metaphor as a means of conceptualizing mental retardation and other disability conditions. Parents who choose to bring an 'impaired' child into the world may increasingly come to be viewed in a similar way to parents who refuse to allow their children to become vaccinated: as purposefully inflicting a potential carrier of disease on the community.

Importantly, the concept that undergirds the organism metaphor, that certain persons pose a risk or threat to the integrity of the community, plays a key role in the psychological reaction that non-disabled persons frequently have to persons with disabilities. As Livneh wrote in his discussion of the origins of pejorative responses to persons with disabilities, in many cases these adverse reactions are largely subconscious in nature, and arise in part from the concern that many non-disabled persons have that contact with disabled individuals indeed does pose a risk to their own bodily integrity or physical or mental well-being.[114]

Various elements of the organism metaphor, such as risk presumption, transmission fears, the need to protect ourselves against the ingestion or invasion of impure substances, and concerns about the degenerative breakdown of our bodies because of such invasion, play a key but subconscious role in the personal decisions we make on a daily basis.[115] It is only natural, therefore, that we should extend such considerations to the larger environment within which we live. I would contend that the frequent utilization of rhetorical elements of the organism metaphor in current social and political dialogue is reinforced by the fact that those who employ such rhetoric understand the important part it plays in our psychological understanding of our world and the transactions between various social groups. Indeed, the organism metaphor may be the principal thematic approach for conceptualizing the status and role of community 'out-groups', as well as for reinforcing restrictive governmental and private policies against such groups.

Notes

1 Sections of this chapter were originally published in the author's 'Protecting the social body: Use of the organism metaphor in fighting the 'menace of the feeble-minded', *Mental Retardation* 37 (1999), 188–200, and 'Social justice implications of the organism metaphor', *Journal of Sociology and Social Welfare* 37 (2010), 95–113.

2 E. Huntington, *Tomorrow's Children: The Goal of Eugenics* (New York: John Wiley & Sons, Inc., 1935), pp. 45–6.

3 D.N. Levine, 'The organism metaphor in sociology', *Social Research* 62 (1995), 239–40; See also Zuckier, 'The essential "other" and the Jew', p. 1112.

4 Levine, 'The organism metaphor in sociology', p. 253. Also see A. Musolff's *Metaphor and Political Discourse: Analogical Reasoning in Debates about Europe* (Palgrave Press, 2004), chapter 5.

5 Musolff, *Metaphor and Political Discourse*, p. 83.

6 Martin Pernick provides an instructive overview of the contagion aspect of the organism metaphor in 'Contagion and culture', *American Literary History* 14 (2002), 858–65.

7 Noël, *Intolerance*, p. 119.

8 For more on Spencer's view of human progress and heredity, see J.D.Y. Peel, *Herbert Spencer: The Evolution of a Sociologist* (New York: Basic Books, Inc., 1971), pp. 144–51.

9 H. Spencer, *The Study of Sociology* (New York: D. Appleton and Company, 1904), p. 301.

10 Levine, 'The organism metaphor in sociology', p. 247. See also E.A. Carlson, *The Unfit: A History of a Bad Idea* (Cold Spring Harbor, NY: Cold Spring Harbor Laboratory Press, 2001), p. 125. Also see English, *Unnatural Selections*, p. 4.

11 G. Chatterton-Hill, *Heredity and Selection in Sociology* (London: Adam and Charles Black, 1907), pp. 257–61.

12 H.P. Fairchild, *Immigration: A World Movement and its American Significance* (New York: Macmillan Company, 1926), p. 398. For contagion and immigrant groups, also see Y. Park and S.P. Kemp, '"Little alien colonies": Representations of immigrants and their neighborhoods in social work discourse, 1875–1924', *Social Service Review* 80 (2006), 705–34.

13 For an extended description of the 'Jewish semen' quotation, see *Nazi Conspiracy and Aggression*, vol. VIII, Office of United States Chief of Counsel for Prosecution of Axis Criminality (Washington, DC: United States Government Printing Office, 1947), p. 12.

14 H. Spencer, *Social Statics*, abridged and rev. version (New York: D. Appleton and Co., 1893), pp. 150–1.

15 See, for example, Harrington, 'Metaphoric connections', p. 373; 'Nazified medi-
    cine', *New York Times* (6 December 1942), section IV, 11; 'New German
    etymology for eugenics', *Eugenical News* 19:5 (1934), 125–6; Proctor, *Racial
    Hygiene*, chapter 3, and *The Nazi War on Cancer* (Princeton, NJ: Princeton
    University Press, 1999); Weindling, *Health, Race and German Politics*, p. 291,
    and Weindling's *Epidemics and Genocide in Eastern Europe, 1890–1945* (Oxford:
    Oxford University Press, 2000), chapters 2 and 3.

16 H.M. Hanauske-Able, 'From Nazi holocaust to nuclear holocaust: A lesson to
    learn'?, *Lancet* 2:8501 (1986), 271–2. Also see A. Musolff, 'What role do meta-
    phors play in racial prejudice? The function of anti-semitic imagery in Hitler's
    Mein Kampf, *Patterns of Prejudice* 41 (2007), 21–43.

17 R.D. Ward, 'The crisis in our immigration policy', *Institution Quarterly* 4:2 (1913),
    37.

18 L. Stoddard, *The Revolt against Civilization: The Menace of the Under Man* (New
    York: Charles Scribner's Sons, 1923), p. 238.

19 In '"Biological Purge" is Urged by Hooton', *New York Times* (21 February 1937),
    section II, 2.

20 S.D. Risley, 'Is asexualization ever justifiable in the case of imbecile children'?,
    Journal of Psycho-Asthenics 9 (1905), 93.

21 M.B. Kirkbride, 'The army of sorrow', *Survey* 26 (1911), 228.

22 Huntington, *Tomorrow's Children*, p. 45.

23 L. Stern, 'Heredity and environment: The Bilder clan', in *Proceedings of the National
    Conference of Social Work* (Chicago: University of Chicago Press, 1922), p. 188.

24 M.W. Barr, 'The imbecile and epileptic *versus* the tax-payer and the community',
    in *Proceedings of the National Conference on Charities and Correction* (Boston: Geo.
    H. Ellis, 1902), p. 163.

25 F.B. Sherbon, 'Eugenics and democracy: Are the two compatible'?, *Eugenics* 2
    (1929), 29.

26 A brief extract from this text is included as the introductory quotation of this
    chapter.

27 A. Holmes, 'Eugenics', *Institution Quarterly* 5 (1914), 158.

28 Stoddard, *The Revolt against Civilization*, pp. 94, 106.

29 'Sterilize the feeble-minded? Pro and con', *Reader's Digest* 32 (May 1938), 98.

30 Sherbon, 'Eugenics and democracy', p. 28.

31 A.E. Wiggam, 'The rising tide of degeneracy: What everyone ought to know about
    eugenics', *World's Work* 53 (November 1926), 26 (italics in original).

32 R.D. Ward, 'Race betterment and our immigration laws', in *Proceedings of the
    First Race Betterment Conference* (Battle Creek, MI: Race Betterment Foundation,
    1914), p. 543.

33 C.B. Davenport, 'The Nams: The feeble-minded as country dwellers', *Survey* 27
    (1912), 1845.

34 C.B. Davenport, 'Report of Committee on Eugenics', *American Breeders Magazine*
    1:2 (1910), 128.

35 M.W. Barr, 'President's annual address', *Journal of Psycho-Asthenics* 2 (1897), 7.

36 Barr, 'The imbecile and epileptic *versus* the tax-payer and the community', p. 163.

37 J.B. Peabody, 'Putting it up to philanthropy' (letter to the editor), *Survey* 29 (1912), 99.

38 S.J. Holmes, *The Eugenic Predicament* (New York: Harcourt, Brace and Company, 1933), p. 101.

39 Goddard, *The Kallikak Family*, p. 71.

40 See, for example, B.T. Baldwin, 'The psychology of mental deficiency', *Popular Science Monthly* 79 (1911), 82; K. Schwartz, 'Nature's corrective principle in social evolution', *Journal of Psycho-Asthenics* 13 (1908), 83; Ward, 'The crisis in our immigration policy', p. 40.

41 B. Van Wagenen, 'Surgical sterilization as a eugenic measure', *Journal of Psycho-Asthenics* 18 (1914), 186.

42 F.L. Sanville, 'Social legislation in the Keystone State: A program in behalf of the mentally unfit', *Survey* 33 (1915), 668.

43 'Pictures the cure for legislative sloth', *Survey* 37 (1917), 725.

44 Nies, *Eugenic Fantasies*, p. 33.

45 'The need for further study of the Piney families', *Eugenical News* 10:6 (1925), 77.

46 Martin Kallikak was supposedly the ancestor who initiated the 'bad' line of Kallikaks. An upstanding citizen himself, according to Goddard he made the mistake of having a brief affair with a presumably feeble-minded bar-maid. She bore a son who was responsible for creating the line that would lead, after multiple generations, to Deborah Kallikak, as well as hundreds of other morons, thieves, drunkards, and prostitutes.

47 Goddard, *The Kallikak Family*, p. 69.

48 M.F. Guyer, *Being Well-Born: An Introduction to Heredity and Eugenics* (Indianapolis: Bobbs-Merrill Company, 1927), p. 347.

49 M.F. Guyer, 'Sterilization', in *Proceedings of the Wisconsin Conference on Charities and Corrections* (Madison: Bobbs-Merrill Company, 1913), p. 46.

50 E.S. Gosney and P. Popenoe, *Sterilization for Human Betterment*, reprint edn. (New York: Macmillan Company, 1980), p. 7.

51 MacMurchy, 'The relation of feeble-mindedness to other social problems', in *Proceedings of the National Conference on Charities and Correction* (Chicago: Hildmann Printing Co., 1916), p. 231.

52 A.W. Butler, 'A notable factor of social degeneracy', *Indiana Bulletin* (December 1901), 18. Also see Butler's 'The burden of feeble-mindedness', in *Proceedings of the National Conference on Charities and Corrections* (Indianapolis: Press of Wm. B. Burford, 1907), p. 2.

53 W.E. Fernald, 'Care of the feeble-minded', in *Proceedings of the National Conference on Charities and Correction* (Press of Fred J. Heer, 1904), p. 383.

54 E. Yukins, 'Feeble-minded white women and the spectre of proliferating perversity in American eugenics narratives', in L.A. Cuddy and C.M. Roche (eds.), *Evolution and Eugenics in American Literature and Culture, 1880–1940: Essays on*

Ideological Conflict and Complicity (Lewisburg, PA: Bucknell University Press, 2003), p. 165.

55 MacMurchy, 'The relation of feeble-mindedness to other social problems', in *Proceedings of the National Conference on Charities and Correction*, p. 232.

56 See, for example, P. Popenoe and R.H. Johnson, *Applied Eugenics* (New York: Macmillan Co., 1933), p. 153.

57 Goddard, *The Kallikak Family*, pp. 73–4.

58 Rafter, *White Trash*, pp. 26–8.

59 E.S. Talbot, *Degeneracy: Its Causes, Signs, and Results*, reprint edn. (New York: Garland Publishing, Inc., 1984), pp. 13–16. For more on the parasite in eugenic writing, see Rafter's *White Trash*, pp. 48–9, 59.

60 Mencken, 'Utopia by sterilization', p. 399.

61 See M.H. Haller, *Eugenic: Hereditarian Attitudes in American Thought* (New Brunswick: Rutgers University Press, 1963), p. 120.

62 Rafter, *White Trash*, p. 17.

63 Kite, 'The "Pineys"', p. 10.

64 Fernald, 'Care of the feeble-minded', p. 388.

65 Stoddard, *The Revolt against Civilization*, p. 233.

66 Sanville, 'Social legislation in the Keystone State', p. 667.

67 N. Deutsch, *Inventing America's 'Worst' Family: Eugenics, Islam, and the Fall and Rise of the Tribe of Ishmael* (Berkeley, CA: University of California Press, 2009), pp. 50–1.

68 C.H. Robinson, 'Toward curbing differential births and lowering taxes, II: Eugenic custody for unfit breeders', *Journal of Heredity* 29 (1938), 260.

69 L.J. Cole, 'The relation of philanthropy and medicine to race betterment', in *Proceedings of the First National Congress on Race Betterment* (Battle Creek, MI: Race Betterment Foundation, 1914), pp. 498–9.

70 Sherbon, 'Eugenics and democracy', p. 28.

71 E.A. Hooton, *Crime and the Man*, reprint edn. (New York: Greenwood Press, 1968), p. 398.

72 Pernick, *The Black Stork*, p. 95 (italics in original).

73 E.R. Johnstone, 'Practical provision for the mentally deficient', in *Proceedings of the National Conference of Charities and Correction* (Fort Wayne, IN: Press of Fort Wayne Printing Co., 1908), p. 316.

74 J. McPhee, *The Pine Barrens*, 2nd edn. (New York: Farrar, Straus, & Giroux, 1968), p. 52.

75 W.E. Fernald, 'The burden of feeble-mindedness', *Journal of Psycho-Asthenics* 17 (1912), 93.

76 S. Humphrey, 'Parenthood and social conscience', *Forum* 49 (1913), 462.

77 W.G. Hague, *The Eugenic Marriage*, vol. I (New York: Review of Reviews Company, 1914), p. 42.

78 Quoted in Trent, *Inventing the Feeble Mind*, p. 143.

79 'Minutes of the Association', *Journal of Psycho-Asthenics* 22 (1917), 22.

80 Pernick, *The Black Stork*, p. 52.

81 J.P Spiro, *Defending the Master Race: Conservation, Eugenics, and the Legacy of Madison Grant* (Burlington, VT: University of Vermont Press, 2009), p. 239.

82 *Buck* decision quoted in Dudziak, 'Oliver Wendell Holmes as a eugenic reformer', p. 858. Also see *Buck v. Bell*, 143 Va. Ct. App. (Keyser-Doherty Printing Co., 1926), pp. 310–24, and Laughlin, 'Further studies on the historical and legal development', p. 101.

83 E.S. Gosney, 'Eugenic sterilization: Human betterment demands it', *Scientific American* 151 (1934), 18–19, 52–3.

84 C.J. Gamble, 'Eugenic sterilization in the United States', *Eugenical News* 34:1–2 (1949), 1.

85 L. Stoddard, *The Rising Tide of Color against White World-Supremacy* (New York: Charles Scribner's Sons, 1922), pp. 159–260. I credit Edwin Black for drawing my attention to this quotation, in his *War against the Weak*, p. 133.

86 O'Brien, 'Indigestible food, conquering hordes', p. 37.

87 C.J. Cannon, 'Selecting citizens' *North American Review* 217 (1923), 325.

88 J.D. Whelpley, 'The overtaxed melting-pot', *Living Age* 281 (1914), 71–2.

89 R.D. Ward, 'Natural eugenics in relation to immigration', *North American Review* 192 (1910), 64.

90 W.E. Fernald, 'What is practical in the way of prevention of mental defect?', in *Proceedings of the National Conference on Charities and Correction* (Chicago: Hildemann Printing Co., 1915), p. 291.

91 W.E. Fernald, 'The feeble-minded', *Educational Review* 54 (1917), 122.

92 Pernick, *The Black Stork*, p. 84.

93 Cole, 'The relation of philanthropy and medicine to race betterment', p. 503.

94 Laughlin quotation in Kühl, *The Nazi Connection*, p. 25.

95 Stoddard, *The Revolt against Civilization*, pp. 245–52.

96 This view was predominant in Germany before to Hitler. See, for example, D. Gasman, *The Scientific Origins of National Socialism: Social Darwinism in Ernst Haeckel and the German Monist League* (New York: American Elsevier Inc., 1971), pp. 91–4; K. Binding and A. Hoche, 'Permitting the destruction of unworthy life: Its extent and form' (1920), trans. W.E. Wright, *Issues in Law and Medicine* 8 (1992), 262. For a very interesting overview of the role of the organism metaphor in Hitler's philosophy, see Musolff's 2007 article 'What role do metaphors play in racial prejudice?'

97 Weindling, *Epidemics and Genocide in Eastern Europe*, pp. 30–2, 43–5.

98 Ibid., p. 45.

99 Hitler, *Mein Kampf*. For examples of Hitler's use of the organism metaphor in the book, see ibid., pp. 30, 57–8, 151, 232–3, 328, 396–8, 440.

100 Musolff, 'What role do metaphors play in racial prejudice?'

101 See, for example, 'New German etymology for eugenics', p. 126; J. Oplinger, *The Politics of Demonology* (Selingsgrove: Sesquehanna University Press, 1990), p. 230; C.B. Cohen, 'The Nazi analogy in bioethics' (commentary), *Hastings*

Center Report 18:5 (1988), 33; R. Altman, 'Selection from the skies' (translation), *Living Age* 357:4477 (1939), 132; Müller-Hill, *Murderous Science*, p. 45; Weindling, *Health, Race and German Politics*, p. 291. Also see the quotation from Konrad Lorenz in A. Chase, *The Legacy of Malthus* (New York: Alfred A. Knopf, 1977), p. 349.

102 'Sterilization law is termed humane', *New York Times* (22 January 1934), 6. Also see Musolff, 'What role do metaphors play in racial prejudice?'

103 Quoted in G. Enderis, 'Reich takes over rights of states', *New York Times* (31 January 1934), 13. Also see Musolff, 'What role do metaphors play in racial prejudice?'

104 G. Fleming, *Hitler and the Final Solution* (Berkeley, CA: University of California Press, 1982), p. 23.

105 Müller-Hill, *Murderous Science*, pp. 97–8.

106 R. Breitman, *The Architect of Genocide: Himmler and the Final Solution* (New York: Alfred A. Knopf, 1991); H. Friedlander, 'From "euthanasia" to the "final solution"', in *Deadly Medicine: Creating the Master Race* (Washington, DC: United States Holocaust Memorial Museum, 2004), p. 182; R. Hilberg, *The Destruction of the European Jews*, reprint edn. (Chicago: Quadrangle Books, 1967), p. 130.

107 Oplinger, *The Politics of Demonology*, pp. 245–6.

108 Müller-Hill, *Murderous Science*, p. 70.

109 Sontag, *Illness as Metaphor*, p. 136. Also see Keen, *Faces of the Enemy*, p. 64.

110 See, for example, G. Aly, P. Chroust, and C. Pross, *Cleansing the Fatherland: Nazi Medicine and Racial Hygiene*, trans. B. Cooper (Baltimore: Johns Hopkins University Press, 1994), pp. 141–2; Hilberg, *The Destruction of the European Jews*, p. 130; M.R. Marrus, *The Unwanted* (Oxford: Oxford University Press, 1985), pp. 228–30; Müller-Hill, *Murderous Science*, pp. 72–3; Office of United States Chief of Counsel for Prosecution of Axis Criminality, *Nazi Conspiracy and Aggression*, vol. V (Washington, DC: United States Government Printing Office, 1947), pp. 334–6.

111 See Aly, Chroust, and Pross, *Cleansing the Fatherland*, p. 49.

112 S. Krugman, J. Giles, and J. Hammond, 'Infectious hepatitis: Evidence for two distinctive clinical, epidemiological and immunological types of infection', *Journal of the American Medical Association* 200 (1967), 95–103; 'Is serum hepatitis only a special type of infectious hepatitis?', *Journal of the American Medical Association* 200 (1967), 136–7. For the radiation experiments, see the United States Department of Energy's *Advisory Committee on Human Radiation Experiments - Final Report* (Washington, DC: U.S. Government Printing Office, 1995), chapter 7.

113 For examples, see D.J. Ingle, *Who Should Have Children?* (Indianapolis: Bobbs-Merrill Co., Inc., 1973), p. 81; W. Shockley, 'Eugenic, or anti-dysgenic, thinking exercises', in R. Pearson (ed.), *Shockley on Eugenics and Race: The Application of Science to the Solution of Human Problems*, reprint edn. (Washington, DC: Scott-Townsend, Publishers, 1992), p. 211; D. Nelkin and L. Tancredi, *Dangerous*

Diagnostics: The Social Power of Biological Information (New York: Basic Books, 1989), p. 13.

114 H. Livneh, 'On the origins of negative attitudes toward people with disabilities', in R. Marinelli and A.D. Dell Orto (eds.), *The Psychological and Social Impact of Disability*, 3rd edn. (New York: Springer Publishing Company, 1991), pp. 181–96.

115 See, for example, Douglas, *Purity and Danger*; Miller, *The Anatomy of Disgust*.

3

THE ANIMAL METAPHOR: THE MORON AS AN ATAVISTIC SUBHUMAN[1]

There is something unnatural about these fellows. Do not listen to their gospel, Señor Commander: it is dangerous. Beware of the pursuit of the Super-human: it leads to an indiscriminate contempt for the Human. To a man, horses and dogs and cats are mere species, outside the moral world. Well, to the Superman, men and women are a mere species too, also outside the moral world.[2]

If the group that is the target for social control can be viewed as falling short of that which defines the fully human, their mistreatment can be justified as in keeping with their quasi- or non-human status. Horst von Maltitz wrote that 'the equating of man and animal' has often 'represented an effort to justify the ruthless treatment' of one's enemies. Such treatment, he noted, is much more socially acceptable when it is directed at 'animalistic' beings than when fellow humans are the targets.[3] According to J. David Smith, Erik Erikson, the famous developmental psychologist,

[H]as attributed inhumane judgments and action by otherwise decent human beings to what he terms *pseudospeciation*. This is how he referred to the process of an 'in' group defining an 'out' group and deciding that its members were less than human. When it is believed that a certain group is not really human, the normal standards of human conduct toward them no longer apply. Therefore, they may be treated in ways that would be unacceptable in the normal course of human relationships.[4]

Animalization is the predominant means of dehumanizing undesirable community members. Principal methods of animalizing a particular group may include the wide-scale dissemination of actual physical, cognitive, or behavioral comparisons between its members and specific animals or the pervasive employment of rhetoric that serves to juxtapose negative animalistic images onto the target group. A debasing cycle may develop, as the treatment of group members in an animalistic fashion often arises when they are perceived as subhuman entities, and such treatment thereupon reinforces the depiction that they indeed are animalistic entities. Thus the reification of the metaphor is somewhat similar to what was discussed in the previous chapter regarding the organism metaphor.

The most basic form of animalization is the employment of animal metaphors as a means of describing the presumptive characteristics of target group members. Animalistic metaphors often highlight the danger that these groups are said to represent. Sam Keen, in *Faces of the Enemy*, provides a number of examples wherein the opposition side was characterized as a threatening rapacious animal within the context of wartime propaganda. Normally, however, even in war, the other is not a 'stronger' animal against which the community or nation must defend itself, as this would indicate weakness on the part of the 'home' nation. Those perceived as enemy combatants are characterized as a threat only because they do not fight fairly or because they 'gang up' or do not confine themselves to the moral standards of 'humane' peoples.[5]

As noted in the previous chapter, marginalized groups have frequently been compared to particularly loathsome and repulsive animals, such as parasites, lice, leeches, termites, bugs, and other vermin.[6] Such animals are so inconsequential from a physical standpoint that their extermination carries with it no guilt for those doing the killing, and on the other hand they can be so destructive or bothersome that their eradication is justified as being not only appropriate but indeed necessary for purposes of community health or protection of one's property. These portrayals symbolize waste, degeneration, and the eating away of that which is healthy and good. As Keen wrote, 'the lower down in the animal phyla the images descend, the greater sanction is given to the soldier [or social control agent] to become a mere exterminator of pests'. He added that '[t]he anti-Semitic propaganda that reduced the Jew to louse or rat was an integral part of the creation of the extermination camps'.[7]

It should be noted that animal metaphors can be used to highlight positive as well as negative attributes of individuals or groups. Because the eagle, for example, symbolizes strength, beauty, independence, vigilance and grace, it does not serve as a 'carrier' of negative meaning, especially in the United States. Nazi propaganda too compared Germany's soldiers to lions: fierce, proud, defenders of the nation. Even small animals such as ants are often used to imply positive qualities such as industry, cooperation, and strength. As the late disability scholar Burton Blatt noted, not only do we anthropomorphize animals, giving them 'human' qualities and characteristics, but we further use these images to support both positive and negative group stereotypes.[8]

The reference to particular animals in denigrating a group is especially apt to occur when specific attributes of the animal in question appear to accurately depict the pejorative stereotypical characteristics of group members, especially those characteristics that underlie or reinforce distancing from and fear of the group. For example, octopi, with their many destructive tentacles, often are used to portray a group that is said to be encroaching into numerous areas of society for the purpose of engaging in sabotage or preparing a take-over of the nation (e.g., communists, Jews). Rats depict filth, disease, and underhandedness, unseen but dangerous groups are often represented by snakes, and rabbits or roaches are frequently used as analogues when the group is accused of rapid procreation.

An additional form of dehumanization is the employment of a hierarchical continuum of humanity based on those characteristics that are accepted as setting humans apart from other animals. Such hierarchical arrangements place a varying degree of value on individuals on the basis of the particular attributes or social status they hold. Inherent in such a structure is the stated fact or assumption that those who are nearest the bottom of the hierarchy are the least human.[9] An important example of this linear hierarchy is the 'Great Chain of Being'. The Chain is a major philosophical construct that has found acceptance in one form or another throughout the ages.[10] It is a vertical scale on which all physical and spiritual entities (e.g., angels, saints, God) have been placed according to their level of perfection, complexity, or perceived valuation. According to Arthur Lovejoy, humans were traditionally viewed as holding a place in the middle of the Chain, since, through our dualistic nature as physical and intellectual beings, we link the 'animalistic' and the 'spiritual' segments of the continuum.[11]

The boundaries which separated one species on the Chain of Being from that above or below it were felt to be fairly obscure. Many advocates of the Chain of Being believed that there was so little difference between the various 'species' within the scale that it was quite difficult to adequately denote the boundaries separating them.[12] This imprecision led to much speculation, especially during the late eighteenth and early nineteenth centuries, as to where the ape, chimpanzee, or orangutan joined with the 'lowest' humans. Many writers thought that these lowest forms of humanity were to be found among the so-called primitive peoples of the globe, whose physical characteristics and mannerisms seemed, at least to these observers, to hearken back to our animalistic past.[13] De Gobineau's early scale of the races included Africans as filling the lowest segment of the hierarchy, as he deemed them to be animalistic and relatively unintelligent.[14] Lovejoy noted that Carolus Linnaeus, creator of the taxonomic scale, 'mentiones a *homo troglodytes*, concerning whom it was not established with certainty whether he was more nearly related to the pygmy or the orang-outang'. He added that the African Hottentots were likely judged among the 'lowest races' in the seventeenth and eighteenth centuries, and that 'more than one writer of the period saw in them a connecting link between the anthropoids and *homo sapiens*'.[15] James Trent described exhibitions at the 1904 St Louis World Fair that presented the members of 'primitive tribes' in environments constructed supposedly to simulate their native habitats. The Philippines exhibit, for example, included a number of tribes whose taxonomic classification either could not be clearly established or was purportedly a link between mankind and our simian ancestors.[16] The idea of the Great Chain of Being, duBois contended, has remained with us for centuries and continues to impact the ways in which we consider differences between various groups.[17] It also has been used to rationalize 'an order in the world in which some beings in the hierarchy dominate others, with a comfortable sense of their innate superiority, given to them "by nature" or by God'.[18]

The beliefs in multiple evolutionary pathways and that some individuals and groups constitute an atavistic throwback to an earlier age both relate closely to this perception of a hierarchical scale of humanity. Obviously the perceived primitivism of the subjected group was an important concept that fostered slavery, actions against Native Americans and other aboriginal groups, imperialism, and many other forms of subjugation. The conquered, it was often argued, could not make their own decisions in a wise manner, were not capable of properly controlling their finances and other resources, needed to be tamed to control their wild nature, and, in a great many ways, were better off and happier in a subservient role. This rationale for social control overlaps with the altruistic metaphor, which will be further discussed in Chapter 5. Among others, Ernst Haeckel in Germany and Louis Agassiz in the United States were both influential in proposing that the various races of humans were progressing along differing evolutionary tracts, with the 'white' races obviously leading the way.[19] As Horsman wrote, the belief in multiple points of human origin and thus differential racial or ethnic 'developmental trajectories' was frequently used to buttress manifest destiny in the United States.[20] While this belief reached its peak decades before the eugenic era, it certainly made its influence felt on the eugenics movement, as will be discussed later in this chapter.

To Cesera Lombroso, the early Italian criminologist, who wrote toward the end of the 1900s, 'born' criminals constituted an atavistic throwback to an earlier, more primitive stage of human evolution. Such atavism, he argued, 'may go back far beyond the savage, even to the brutes themselves'.[21] To Lombroso, born criminals resembled 'lemurs and rodents' in some respects. Epileptics too, he noted, many of whom he classified as criminalistic, possessed many of the characteristics of 'instinctive animalism'.[22] According to Lombroso, these primitive traits could be found primarily among members of the lower classes. He further believed that since such atavism was largely hereditary and unalterable, punishment – or any other form of treatment, for that matter – would have little rehabilitative effect on 'born criminals'. The only appropriate social response was therefore to find such persons early and segregate them from the rest of the community.[23] Francis Galton too spoke of criminals as atavistic, writing that '[a] man who is counted as an atrocious criminal in England, and is punished as such by English law in social self-defence, may nevertheless have acted in strict accordance with instincts that are laudable in less civilised societies'.[24]

Throughout history, scapegoats of all types have been viewed as chimerical beings possessing both human and animal traits. Entities that defy categorization have always evoked feelings of both wonder and defilement, conjuring up at the same time visions of awe and mystery alongside those of trepidation and fear. Infants too have often been perceived as holding quasi-human status. In various cultures the killing of a child was acceptable until he or she reached a particular stage of development. This was frequently one way of ensuring that child who had disability conditions that were not observable at birth would not live to reach adulthood.[25] Even in contemporary discussions of passive or active euthanasia, many have argued that allowing – or, in some cases, assisting – newborns to die is less morally problematic than bringing about the deaths of older children or adults.

The animalization of 'feeble-minded' persons prior to the eugenic era

Of all marginalized groups, surely those with severe cognitive impairments are among the most vulnerable to being animalized. The taxonomic status of persons with mental disabilities, especially mental retardation, has been a topic of intense debate for centuries.[26] Even before 1900 Alice Mott noted that in many cultures idiots had been classified as brutes or animals.[27] In 1873 the British physician Henry Maudsley wrote that in some persons the brain stopped short of its full human development, and 'remains arrested at or below the level of an orang[utan]'s brain'.[28] He shared one particular case, originally described by the 'Deputy Commissioner in Lunacy for Scotland', who said that he had never

> seen a better illustration of the ape-faced idiot than in this case. It is not, however, the face alone that is ape-like. He grins, chatters, and screams like a monkey, never attempting a sound in any way resembling a word. He puts himself in the most ape-like attitude in his hunts after lice, and often brings his mouth to help his hands.[29]

In 1898 Eugene Talbot, a Chicago oral surgeon with a particular interest in the nature of human degeneration, wrote that '[w]ith the brain of the orang type comes a corresponding defect of function. With this animal type of brain in idiocy sometimes appear animal traits and instincts'.[30] Margaret Bancroft added that 'Vogt, a disciple of Darwin, thought characteristics of the microcephalic patient resembled those of the anthropoid ape'.[31] According to Talbot, Vogt believed that in some cases the brains of idiots were much less evolved than this, and similar to those found in reptiles and birds.[32]

As described above, public fascination with the missing link and those humans who seemingly provided a connection with our atavistic ancestors grew extensively throughout the second half of the nineteenth century, especially after publication of Darwin's *On the Origin of Species*.[33] The use of persons with microcephaly and other forms of intellectual disabilities in carnival sideshows as missing links or 'monkey-men' compelled the public to question whether such entities could be considered fully human. One of the more famous of these 'wild-men' had a 'keeper' and was exhibited in a cage for much of his career. While he actually hailed from New Jersey, he was said to have been found by a group of African explorers, who 'came upon a group of this race that had never before been seen'. According to Robert Bogdan, this mysterious tribe was advertised as having been found 'in a "perfectly nude state"', and moved 'through the trees and their branches like monkeys and orangutangs'.[34] 'The association of various human differences with danger, inferiority, subhuman characteristics, and animal traits', Bogdan contended, 'was developed as well as perpetuated by these exhibits.'[35]

Another relevant construct that had a long history in European folklore, but continued through the Enlightenment, was the changeling. The changeling was a quasi-human animal that was believed to have been left (by evil spirits, trolls, etc.) in place of a human child. The belief in the changeling was frequently used to rationalize the birth of a mentally disabled child. As Goodey noted, the famous philosopher John Locke, among others, perceived idiots or changelings to be have a physical nature similar to humans, but to lack rational thought, and thus souls.[36] As discussed below, questions about whether persons with intellectual disabilities could be counted as rational beings, and, if not, where they fell on the line from human to animal, carried over into and even beyond the eugenic era.

The historical role of the feeble-minded person as an animalistic source of amusement is also evidenced by the institutional practice of charging visitors an admission price to gawk at and ridicule residents. Until the eighteenth century, a number of facilities serving persons who had been categorized as insane or feeble-minded, most notably Bethlem in London, but also some

American hospitals and asylums, supplemented their income this way.[37] Reformers from Dorothea Dix to Michel Foucault have described the animalistic treatment of persons labeled as insane and idiotic within both institutional and community settings.[38]

Public interest in those entities that seem to fall within the border separating the human and the non-human can also be seen in the centuries-old lore of feral children. Pierre-Joseph Bonnaterre, for example, one of the first professionals to study Victor, the 'Wild Boy of Aveyron', wrote that 'if it were not for his human face, what would distinguish him from the apes?' Victor, Bonnaterre continued, 'is truly and purely an animal ... what enormous barriers separate him from us!' Even the renowned reformer Philippe Pinel viewed Victor as little removed from the realm of non-human animals. Throughout his study of the boy, which is quoted in Harlan Lane's *The Wild Boy of Aveyron*, Pinel compares Victor (mostly unfavorably) to wild and domesticated animals, and he repeatedly talks about the boy's 'animal instinct'.[39] As Lane pointed out, seminal questions about the nature of the human that were central to the Enlightenment, such as the relative importance of nature and nurture and the potential impact of education, especially on groups that were perceived to be primitive, were inextricably connected to the efforts of Pinel and others to 'humanize' Victor. While these questions were still up for discussion in the United States during the middle part of the nineteenth century, by the end of the century most professionals had come to agree that education and training would do very little to bring persons with intellectual disabilities into the sphere of humanity.[40]

The belief in maternal impressions was yet another example of the way in which animalistic elements were juxtaposed onto children with impairments, although this related to those with physical disabilities more than to those with mental disabilities. The core feature of this belief was that pregnant women could be so affected by certain disgusting, highly disconcerting, or violent visual images that these images, or the trauma caused by them, could impact the development and appearance of their unborn children. Prior to the turn of the century, expectant women were often warned to stay away from carnival side-shows, for example, for fear that what they viewed would form a permanent disfiguring impression on their child.[41] As early as the 1600s François Bayle wrote that the 'nervous juices' of the mother could impact the development of the child so that 'a human foetus may be changed into a monkey in the womb'.[42] Into the twentieth century, popular belief maintained, even among many parents of disabled children, that at least some disability conditions were the result of maternal impressions.[43] In the 1916 biennial report of the State Home for the Feeble-Minded in Winfield, Kansas, the various suspected causes of 'imbecility' in the inmates who were admitted during the period were noted. Ten cases were attributed to maternal impressions.[44]

Eugenics and animalization of the moron

Built on the concept of animal breeding, eugenics by its very nature carried with it an undercurrent of animalization. American eugenicists, as well as their colleagues in other countries, frequently described their goals by drawing comparisons between human and animal breeding.[45] John Kellogg, the physician, health enthusiast, cereal manufacturer, and eugenicist, decried the fact that '[w]e have registries for horses, cattle, sheep, pigs, and even cats and dogs … But nowhere on earth, so far as the writer knows, is there to be found a registry for human thoroughbreds.'[46] Livestock breeders had produced, he noted, 'many varieties of thoroughbred livestock which, in some cases, are possessed of such superior and remarkable characteristics as to virtually constitute new species'.[47] 'Man', he continued, 'has improved every useful creature and every useful plant with which he has come in contact – with the exception of his own species.'[48] Other eugenicists added that we 'face complacency in our own families that we would not tolerate in our piggery',[49] and that '[i]ncreasing the proportion of productive citizens is as simple as raising chickens; first select, preserve and improve the good; second eliminate the bad'.[50] Henry Goddard, in discussing adoption, warned potential adoptive parents that they must take care to ensure the health of their child. He compared parents who did not to a careless farmer who is offered a calf to add to his herd, and accepts the offer without first 'inquir[ing] into the pedigree of that calf, and ascertain[ing] as far as possible what the likelihood was that it would be worth raising'.[51] Moreover, a number of supporters of eugenics, including Alexander Graham Bell, had developed an interest in human breeding in part through their personal experiences with animal husbandry.[52]

Animalistic metaphors and pejorative comparisons with animals were frequently invoked during the eugenic era for the purpose of describing the 'moron' population. W. Duncan McKim, for example, said such persons were 'beings with less intelligence than the goose, with less decency than the pig'.[53] Stern invoked the 'octopus' metaphor, writing that morons 'form a secret sort of community in the neighborhoods in which they live – a secret community spreading out its tentacles and thriving lustily after its own fashion'.[54] In an interesting if highly patronizing animal metaphor, Leon Whitney, the Executive Secretary of the American Eugenics Society, said that generations ago the nation had kindly decided to 'adopt' its feeble-minded citizens in much the same way as someone might take in a 'cute little harmless' stray bear cub. Over time, however, the animal had grown into a menacing beast, and now it had actually begun attacking society.[55] The animals that were primarily compared to the moron in eugenic writings were parasites and the great apes. Examples of the former were provided in the previous Chapter, and the latter will be further discussed below.

Charles Davenport, the leader of the eugenics movement in the United States, frequently spoke of the 'unfit' segment of the population as being more like animals than like humans. Following is one example:

> We are horrified by the 223 capital offenses in England less than a century ago, but though capital punishment is a crude method of grappling with the difficulty it is infinitely superior to that of training the feeble-minded and criminalistic and then letting them loose upon society and permitting them to perpetuate in their offspring these animalistic traits ... If we are to build up in America a society worthy of the species *man* then we must take such steps as will prevent the increase or even the perpetuation of animalistic strains.[56]

In other works he contended that 'in some way or other society must end these animalistic blood-lines or they will end society',[57] and that 'by the elimination of the worst matings of the animalistic strains and by the union of sense and sentiment in many others a more uniform innate capacity in our people may be achieved'.[58]

The absence of reason

The perception that feeble-minded persons were subhuman beings was reinforced by the notion that they lacked 'inborn intelligence' and any semblance of reason. As the following quotation demonstrates, it is often taken to be intelligence that demarcates humans from other animals:

> When into a house for the first time comes the heavenly visitor, father and mother bend over the little body and scan it from head to foot for some physical defect. Happy are they if the child is physically perfect. It is all that it can be. They are satisfied.
>
> By and by come the dawning time of intelligence. Faint sparks of the human begin to gleam through the merely physical activities of their precious little animal.[59]

Unlike persons with chronic mental illness, persons who were feeble-minded had, most eugenicists maintained, no chance to become fully functioning humans. While those who presumably 'lost' their mental capacity could possibly rediscover it, at least partly, those who never had a 'properly functioning' mind in the first place were beyond hope.[60]

Eugenicists assured their readers that, like animals, morons were guided completely by instinct rather than rational thought. Since many believed, as Wright contended, that '[t]he mind is the measure of the man', it naturally followed that those with lesser minds were lesser persons.[61] The 'animal instincts', 'animal passions', or 'animal natures' of feeble-minded persons were a frequent topic of discussion in eugenic literature.[62] The instinctual nature of morons and other 'defectives' was often depicted through animalistic comparisons. Charles Davenport's wife Gertrude wrote in an article that hereditary criminals 'can no more help committing crime than race horses can help going',[63] and Henry Goddard said that feeble-minded women could 'no more live in accordance with the conventions of society than the cats and dogs in the street'.[64] Charles Powlison added that it was mainly the ability to exercise 'control and choice in regard to our instinctive actions' that 'differentiates man from the other animals'.[65]

It naturally followed that since feeble-minded persons were believed to be incapable of controlling their base instincts, it was not easy to differentiate them from non-human animals. Michael Guyer wrote that since it was 'a late acquisition of the race and less firmly ingrained, the social instinct is not well established in all individuals. Some have it sufficiently strong to exercise of their own accord the necessary inhibitions of other instincts ... it is in just these very inhibitions that mental defectives are lacking.'[66] Since feeble-minded persons could not exercise such control, eugenicists contended, they required a degree of external control that other humans did not.

Because they had neither reason nor the capacity to develop it, some argued that, as with 'born' criminals, efforts to educate and reform feeble-minded persons were a waste of time and resources.[67] While morons and other degenerates were said to pose a real threat to society, they were presented by eugenic writers as not responsible for the harm they might cause, because of both their inborn weaknesses and their inability to change. Rather than benefitting members of the group by displacing 'blame' for their condition from them, the primary impact of this perception was to reinforce the argument that they should be brought under social control since they could not be reformed.[68] 'As well try to cure a fox of eating chickens', Goddard wrote, describing the delinquent moron, 'as to attempt to reform such as these by prison sentences, education, or social uplift.'[69] Charles Davenport added that society should treat 'the misdemeanant as we treat a puppy whose actions displease us. Either train him carefully, if he is trainable; otherwise, put him in a position where the exercise of his instincts will not offend us.'[70]

Institutional placement, many argued, was beneficial to the feeble-minded themselves. For outside the segregated environment, they were lazy and shiftless, usually unemployed, and dependent upon the community. In the residential facility, however, they could be trained to work. As laborers, morons were often perceived as 'beasts of burden', capable of doing the hard but non-intellectual work required for efficient operation of the institution. In the writings of eugenicists and many early institutional administrators, the training of the moron often seemed to take on the guise of domestication.[71] One eugenicist argued that simple repetitive labor training was the only type of education appropriate for morons, as 'they were only capable of performing work that they have already learned after painstaking training in much the same way that an animal is taught tricks'.[72]

The deprivation of sensory capacity

Often a presumed lack of sensory acuity among target group members has been employed to depict them as not fully human. Truly human entities, it is argued, experience 'normal' sensory reactivity. They respond adversely to overly hot or cold temperatures and other discomforting sensations, and are especially responsive to painful stimuli. Toward the end of the 1800s Cesare Lombroso wrote that 'born criminals' were relatively 'insensible to pain' and experienced a 'dullness of the sense of touch'.[73] Lombroso quoted an earlier writer who stated that because 'fineness of feeling diminishes in proportion as one descends the social scale, it is not necessary to visit savage peoples; it is enough to talk with the English poor, or even with one's own servants'.[74]

A number of eugenicists spoke of feeble-minded persons as lacking sensation, and this deficiency was often presented as a primary source of support for the moron's status as a 'diminished' human. Before the turn of the century, Alice Mott wrote that '[i]mbeciles after once experiencing the joys of having a tooth extracted will often beg in heart-rending accents for a renewal of the pleasure',[75] and Henry Goddard took note of the fact that, in one of the homes visited as part of the Kallikak study, there was no fire to warm the 'thinly clad' mother and child, and yet '[t]hey did not shiver, however, nor seem to mind'.[76]

When attempting to develop a workable intelligence test, first Francis Galton and later Alfred Binet focused on sensory measures as potentially correlated to general intelligence. As Galton noted in his book *Inquiries into Human Faculty and its Development*, he arrived at this belief in large part because of his observation that idiots 'hardly distinguish between heat and cold, and their sense of pain is so obtuse that some of the more idiotic seem hardly to know what it is'. He further wrote that in the 'dull lives' of idiots, 'such pain as can be excited in them may literally be accepted with a welcome surprise'.[77] Galton provided specific examples to describe why he felt that a relationship existed between intelligence and sensory acuity. Regarding his visit to Earlswood Asylum, near London, he wrote:

> I saw two boys whose toe-nails had grown into the flesh and had been excised by the surgeon. This is a horrible torture to ordinary persons, but the idiot lads were said to have shown no distress during the operation; it was not necessary to hold them, and they looked rather interested at what was being done. I also saw a boy with the scar of a severe wound on his wrist; the story being that he had first burned himself slightly by accident, and, liking the keenness of the new sensation, he took the next opportunity of repeating the experience, but, idiot-like, he overdid it.[78]

Importantly, this perceived diminished sensory acuity can also presuppose a lack of suffering. Elizabeth Kite, the eugenic field worker who investigated the Kallikaks, stated that '[s]uffering comes only with intelligence'.[79] The Germans Binding and Hoche, in their 1920 treatise in support of euthanasia that would influence the Nazis, similarly wrote that '"[s]ympathy" is the last emotional response which is relevant to the life or death of a mentally dead person; where there is no suffering (*Leiden*) there can be no sympathy (*Mit-Leiden*)'.[80] Martin Pernick, in discussing the Bollinger baby infanticide case, which garnered headlines nationally during the eugenic era, noted that, to many eugenicists, 'Not only did defectives lack the ability to suffer, they lacked the capacity for life at all.' He quoted Harry Haiselden, the physician in the case, as declaring 'that the Bollinger baby's "tiny brain ... was not a live thing – but a dead and fearsome ounce or two of jelly ... those who have no brains – their blank and awful existence cannot be called Life ... We live through our brains."'[81]

The moron and hierarchical notions of the human species

A central conceptual metaphor that characterized the eugenics movement was the belief that the human species could be viewed along a hierarchical scale, with placement on the scale being based largely on individual or group characteristics such as intelligence. Of morons, Henry Goddard wrote that '[t]hey are at the lower end of the scale, just as the genius is at the upper end and they differ from the average man just as the genius differs, but in the opposite direction'.[82] Much of the writing of eugenicists conveyed this idea of a simplistic vertical ordering of humans. For example, those who were targeted for eugenic control were often described as the 'submerged tenth' of the population.[83] Another clear example of this verticality is the following, from H.L. Mencken:

> The one and only remedy is to strike at the source of all incompetence, whether social or economic, mental or physical. Let a resolute attack be made upon the

fecundity of *all* the males on the lowest rungs of the racial ladder, and there will be a gradual and permanent improvement.[84]

As in historical precursors such as the Great Chain of Being, described above, some eugenicists saw the 'lower end' of the species hierarchy as grading over into the category populated by the great apes. Charles Davenport was particularly outspoken in this regard. In 1912, for example, he contended that '[t]here are persons who range in intellectual capacity all the way from the most effective and the most cultured to those who have less intelligence than many apes'.[85] Margaret Sanger wrote that society allowed defectives to 'descend to a plane of living below the animal level'.[86] In his observation of a German sterilization court proceeding, the American eugenicist Lothrop Stoddard noted that the first subject he saw 'looked like an excellent candidate for sterilization', citing his observation that the man 'was rather ape-like in appearance'.[87] As noted above, a number of eugenicists echoed the theme that had been long expressed, even before Darwin, that it was the intellect that allowed humans to rise beyond the purely animal. It naturally followed that those humans who did not exhibit intelligence might be fundamentally closer to the great apes than to Homo sapiens. According to Michael Burleigh, in the Nazis' graphic presentations of families with 'deviant offspring', created to demonstrate the large number of children in such families, these persons are depicted as somewhat 'simian' in appearance, since 'the agenda here involved disputing the human personality of the people concerned'.[88]

Possibly the most extraordinary juxtaposition of the moron and the simian appeared in the *Literary Digest* during World War I. This article cited a recently published *Medical Times* editorial recommending that feeble-minded persons be employed on the front lines of battle, since their lives were least valuable, and they could be taught to engage in 'the brutish side of war'. In response to the possible retort that this suggestion was immoral, the author asked whether the employment of apes in a similar way would 'be revolting to the moral sense.' The article then asked whether such use of 'an anthropoid [is] any more objectionable ... than a low-grade imbecile.' 'If we must have war', the piece concluded, 'let us set only the beasts and subnormal men upon each other'.[89] The author who is quoted, Dr Arthur Jacobson, may have been writing satirically. Regardless of the seriousness of the suggestion, however, his union of morons and apes touched on a prevalent cultural theme.

The simian-like nature of morons was also cultivated by writings that presented them as atavistic pre-humans. Some held that since intelligence was a relatively recent evolutionary development in humans it had not been firmly engrained in all 'stocks', as was demonstrated by the births of morons and other defectives.[90] Early in the century George Keene wrote that it was with 'the feeble-minded, the epileptic and the insane' that we truly understand 'the meaning of such terms as "atavistic tendencies", and "reversion to the original type"'.[91] In *The Black Stork*, Martin Pernick noted that Harry Haiselden believed that persons with disabilities, especially when they were born of parents who appeared 'normal', might be 'a throw-back to the darkest jungle days'.[92] Just as some children bore a resemblance to their grandparents, great-grandparents, or even more remote ancestors, in very rare cases it was thought that the genetic traits of a child could embody a more distant, primitive stage in the family's evolutionary history. Of course, it was reasonable to assume then that those parents who were themselves closest to this earlier evolutionary period could most easily imbue their child with such atavistic traits.

To follow up on the discussion of contagion in Chapter 2, some eugenicists utilized animal or breeding metaphors to describe the degenerating impact that morons and others could have on 'good' families. One, for example, said that 'even a single drop of "cur blood" ruined good breeding stock among humans just as it did for animals', and that efforts at 'cross-breeding' served only to 'produce "worthless mongrels"'.[93] The 'mongrel' was a favored metaphor for those eugenicists who opposed miscegenation or even intermarriage between those in different social classes.

Charles Davenport, following the lead of Francis Galton and Cesare Lombroso, contended that a primary feature of both feeble-minded persons and criminals was that they were mistakes of nature whose aptitudes were suited to a previous period in the development of the species when neither morality nor intelligence was a core requisite for social relations or survival. The qualities of such persons, Davenport wrote, 'are unfortunate traits for a twentieth-century citizen but they constitute a first-rate mental equipment for our remote ape-like ancestors'. Many of their behaviors, he continued, 'are crimes for a twentieth-century citizen but they are the normal acts of our remote, ape-like ancestors'.[94] One writer said that trying mentally defective criminals in the court system was similar to practices in some 'earlier cultures that tried animals'. Since such criminals 'were defective, and could not change their ways', they needed to be kept away from society.[95]

Like some other early eugenicists, Davenport believed in recapitulation. This theory held that while feeble-minded persons may have started down the road to becoming 'fully developed', mature humans, something happened to permanently thwart their progress and to keep them lower on the developmental hierarchy than other members of the species. According to this theory, the formation of individuals paralleled the evolutionary development of the species, such that each person, as he or she matured from a fetus to infancy and

to adulthood, advanced through the same stages of growth that the species as
a whole had progressed through during its evolutionary course. Davenport
contended that recapitulation provided an apt description for the status of
feeble-minded persons:

> we may infer that man's remote ancestors did not go in their adult stage beyond
> the point where this infant-man is now. Indeed, the adult apes, nearest allies of
> our ancestors, show the same inability to talk, to dress, to regard property rights
> and to be gentle and considerate toward others that the infant shows. And we
> can not escape the conclusion that the gradual acquisition of social traits by
> the normal child follows much the same road as the evolution of social man
> from non-gregarious apes. But, there are men who never develop these social
> traits. And if we study the pedigrees of such men carefully ... we trace back a
> continuous trail of the defects until the conclusion is forced upon us that the
> defects of this germ plasm have surely come all the way down from man's ape-
> like ancestors, through 200 generations or more ... Feeble-mindedness is, thus,
> an uninterrupted transmission from our animal ancestry. It is not reversion; it is
> direct inheritance.[96]

Many of those who discussed the ape-like status of morons and other
'defectives' noted that their unrestrained child-bearing was weighing down
the forward progression of the species. An important component of the
race suicide argument was the belief, prevalent during the eugenic age, in
the 'degeneration' of the species. Many writers agreed with Francis Galton's
contention that the human species had been on a downward spiral since the
days of the ancient Athenians and Romans. While our technological abilities
had certainly increased, Galton asserted, there was not a concomitant expansion in the bodily structure or mental capacity of humans. Albert Wiggam,
John Kellogg, Earnest Hooton, and other eugenicists wrote in fearful tones of
degeneration,[97] with the latter, for example, quoted in the New York Times as
saying that '[m]an, his physique and behavior, would give to a visiting committee of anthropoid apes a shock and a feeling of satisfaction that their own
system of life was superior'.[98] Another New York Times article about the views
of Hooton, a Harvard anthropology professor, was titled 'Hooton finds man
reverting to ape'.[99]

The moron as a quasi-human or primitive entity

Eugenical descriptions of feeble-minded persons often highlighted their status
as entities that could not quite be considered fully human. The list of quasi-
human terms that were used in eugenic writings to portray morons and other
'defectives' was indeed quite long. Various writers referred to them as 'half-

formed thing[s]' and 'semi-human automata', 'by-products of unfinished humanity', 'half-alive beings', and 'poor-sub-human things', '[h]orrid semi-humans', 'low ember[s]', 'fragments of humanity', 'fragmentary creature[s]', 'bits of defective humanity', 'empty human shells', 'burned-out human husks', and 'minus elements'.[100] The Chicago Judge Harry Olson decried the 'The menace of the half-man',[101] and George Knight, an early institutional admin-istrator, said that even after adequate services had been provided for a feeble-minded resident, the best one could hope for him was that he would be 'two-thirds of a man'.[102] To many eugenicists, morons constituted hybrid entities that included some human characteristics, but not enough to earn them the rights that were due to other humans. Raymond Pearl's statement in support of Dr Haiselden's decision to refuse to treat the Bollinger baby was typical of the belief that morons were doomed to a life as subhumans. In this published letter, Pearl said that the decision was wise since the child 'could never develop into anything even approaching a normal human being'.[103]

As noted in the previous chapter, to some eugenicists, the primitive envi-ronments in which morons lived seemed to provide strong evidence that they could not be considered to be 'fully human' entities. The family studies and other case examples not only described the dwellings of their subjects as primitive, but often added that if they were placed in 'nice' environments or neighborhoods, they would quickly resort to their old ways of living. Members of the 'Tribe of Ishmael', the name given by the author to the subjects of one of the family studies, were said 'to live in hollow trees or the river bottoms',[104] and the Bilder clan, another such family, dwelt 'on the dumps of South Philadelphia in shacks'.[105] Elizabeth Kite noted that the 'Pineys', a family she studied, were, like animals, 'known to penetrate deeper into the woods as civi-lizing influences approach'.[106] Amos Butler described a similar moron couple who lived in the woods and 'were said to make a bed of leaves or straw and live on what they can beg, supplemented by wild fruits and nuts'.[107]

As Nicole Rafter wrote in *White Trash*, animalistic images were frequently included within the eugenic family studies, as 'the cacogenic "mate" and "migrate", "nesting" with their "broods" in caves and "hotbeds where human maggots are spawned"'.[108] She added also that many of the families were 'located in forests, long associated in imaginative literature with mystery, danger, and the illicit'.[109] Rafter concluded that such images not only suggest danger; 'they also imply that the cacogenic would hardly notice if they were treated as less than human'.[110]

Arthur Estabrook's 1913 article entitled 'A two-family apartment', which was published in the *Survey*, a major social reform publication, provided a clear example of the animalistic environmental context within which eugenic writing often placed the rural feeble-minded family. One family, which the author said was descended from the original Jukes, had 'moved into [a] barn-like building', which it shared with a number of pigs (the second 'family' in the article's title). 'The walls of the room', he continued, 'have been covered with wrapping paper, behind which rats can be heard scurrying about ... Filth abounds everywhere, the two families rivals in this respect, the humans being slightly in the lead.'[111]

As quasi-human entities, morons were said to not have the full measure of morality that one would expect to find in 'truly' human beings. This was primarily evidenced, as one might guess, by their supposedly persistent and uncontrolled procreation. 'Many of these people', Mary Kostir wrote in her eugenic family study *The Family of Sam Sixty*, 'are as irresponsible sexually as are rabbits or guinea pigs'.[112] Lothrop Stoddard wrote that feeble-minded persons were 'ever-multiplying swarms of degenerates', and that when they were 'no longer permitted to breed like lice, the floods of chaos will soon dry up'.[113]

As noted in the previous chapter, the frequent reference not only to small insects but also to bacterial growths and related metaphors was in part an effort to demonstrate the rapid breeding of such persons. In response to proposals such as marriage restriction laws, Walter Hadden contended that it would make as much sense to try to 'control the mating of rabbits or mice by legislation'.[114] Rabbits were, as one might assume, a favored metaphor for describing the procreative capacity of feeble-minded persons, especially when the topic of restrictive marriage legislation arose. According to Charles Davenport:

> Some years ago some rabbits were introduced into Australia, and these rabbits multiplied tremendously and overran the country. Now, I can imagine an Australian lawmaker securing the passage of a law to the effect that these rabbits shall not breed any more, thus helping to solve the problem of the destruction of the country by rabbits. This law is about as sensible as a law against the reproduction of defectives or the laws against incest.[115]

Animal metaphors and euthanasia

Animal and subhuman metaphors were particularly apt to be found in the writings of the small number of American eugenicists who openly supported euthanasia as a eugenic method. These writers contended that death would be a blessing to 'humans' who lived such pitiful lives. Foster Kennedy, the leader of the American euthanasia movement before World War II, argued that we needed to treat human beings who were suffering great pain with the same compassion that we would show for a 'stricken horse', and should assist them in dying.[116]

Others frequently questioned the humanity of feeble-minded and other seriously disabled persons. One wrote that 'congenital idiots are monsters, the result of some slip of the hand of Him who made them; lumps of matter in human form but without human mind'.[117] The description of such individuals, especially infants, was often animalistic. Maynard Shipley, a California-based scientist and supporter of eugenics, upon visiting the children's unit of a hospital, wrote that '[i]n the baby ward, where queer misshapen little creatures lay in rows of cots, the attendant lifted from its pillow a tiny bit of flesh that stared with fishy eyes'.[118] To the Germans Binding and Hoche, sympathy for the feeble-minded was 'based on the same inescapable conceptual error ... which leads most people to project their own thoughts and feelings into other living things'. These authors went on to note that '[t]his error also provides one source for the excesses of the European animal rights movement'.[119]

Animalistic descriptions of the lives that feeble-minded and insane persons supposedly lived were disseminated by the Nazis for the purpose of justifying the sterilization program and building public support for euthanasia. Lifton wrote that the cases described by Hitler as indicative of subnormal humanity included institutionalized persons who could '"only be bedded on sand or sawdust because they continually befouled themselves", and in which "patients put their own excrement into their mouths, eating it and so on"'.[120] Examples like these served to buttress the argument that these persons would be better off dead than living such useless lives. As Michael Burleigh wrote in his book *Death and Deliverance*, the Nazis created a number of documentary films to illustrate the 'animalistic' lives that these persons were 'forced to live'. According to Burleigh, in 'some of these films they [the residents of institutions] are explicitly situated a considerable way below the level occupied by animals, who are invariably depicted with greater affection and sensitivity'.[121] These films showed a hand-picked group of the most severely disabled persons, dressed down for the occasion and shown in sinister, dark lighting. They engaged in behaviors that, when not manifestly animalistic, were certainly thought to be uncharacteristic of human beings. Additionally, because of the presumed animalistic status of morons, the Nazis believed that they neither appreciated nor required 'nice' environments in which to live. Even before the euthanasia program began, many residents were moved out of 'attractive' asylums to be replaced by elderly citizens or orphans, who 'would better appreciate these resplendent surroundings'.[122]

Numerous writers have contended that institutionalization itself, both during and since the eugenic era, has often served as a form of 'backdoor euthanasia'.[123] This is not to say that all residential environments, or even most, have fallen into this category. But many institutions, at least, not only have treated their charges as 'animal-like', but have allowed their facilities to bring their charges to an early death, especially through environmentally caused disease. Martin Pernick wrote that Harry Haiselden justified his refusal to treat disabled newborns by citing the 'horrors of institutionalization' from which he was saving them.[124] According to Martin Elks, many institutional officials believed that high mortality rates resulting from tuberculosis and other diseases – or 'lethal selection',[125] as some referred to it – were due to:

> an inherited susceptibility to the disease and that such 'natural selection' would lead to race betterment in the long run. At least some institutions for 'the feebleminded' may thus have functioned as de facto and acceptable locations for 'euthanasia' by providing environments conducive to infectious diseases to which many residents succumbed.[126]

Discussion

Animalization is perhaps the most frequently employed metaphor theme for fostering the devaluation of marginalized human beings. Even the term 'marginalize' relates to groups who stand on the brink of – or even over – a socially constructed boundary-line that demarcates which members of the species are to be provided with meaningful respect, freedom, consideration, or rights. The implications of the quasi-human or non-human status that has traditionally been imposed upon target groups are, then, abundantly clear, even if the audience that responds to such metaphors is only subconsciously aware of them. If persons are not 'authentic' humans, or their 'personhood' can be effectively challenged, they do not have to be treated as full members of the human community. In some cases, moreover, they may be treated with less regard and provided with fewer rights than certain (especially 'useful' or 'productive') animals. Perhaps one of the most disconcerting contradictions of Nazi Germany is that at the same time as prisoners were being worked to death, Jews were being transported to concentration camps in horrendously overcrowded cattle cars, and 'hereditarily disabled' persons were being killed to 'relieve their suffering', policies were being implemented to expand animal rights. As Sax noted, German policies limited the amount of work that could be required of draft and farm animals, provided strict guidelines for the humane transport of animals, limited their involvement in medical experimentation, and set harsh penalties for any form of cruel treatment.[127]

Conceptually, at least, some version of a simplistic vertical ordering of humans has typified virtually all large-scale prejudice-fueled movements of the past, and continues in contemporary discussions about human rights. In many cases this vertical ordering has been characterized by a racial hierarchy dominated by the class of persons who created it. As Gould noted, intelligence testing, too, was in a sense a bastardized update of the Great Chain of Being.[128] By ranking individuals on a hierarchical scale based on one nebulous component, intelligence, eugenicists were able to demonstrate which persons were closest to the modern version of the eugenic icon, and which were furthest from this ideal. An important assumption here, again, is that those who create the scale are quite certain of their own place on it.

In considering various alarm periods, then, social construction is important not only in looking at the specific ways in which groups are described, and thus the rationales that are employed to support social control, but also in delineating bedrock values that support determinations of individual worth. The reason why intelligence became the foundational value of American eugenicists relates largely to the cultural context within which the movement prospered. Indeed, eugenics in Nazi Germany had a substantially different flavor than that in the United States, as the Nazis focused heavily on both physical and intellectual fitness in creating the 'perfect Aryan'. While those who were deemed to be morons were targets of control in Germany, so were many of those on the other end of the 'scale', the so-called intelligentsia.

The middle position which the human species was thought to occupy on the Great Chain of Being is significant. As noted, it has often been contended that humanity is linked to its brutish past, and the anthropoids from which we evolved, by means of the 'lowest' humans. Conversely, the spiritual realm may be seen as connecting with Homo sapiens by way of the 'highest', or most intellectual, insightful, or moral members of the species. Inherent in this philosophy, as many have viewed it over time, is a belief that the species has evolved from its material or animalistic origins, and is continuing to evolve toward a more spiritual plane of existence. We will, it follows, at some future date throw off the physical shackles which have bound us to our material bodies, and join the ranks of the angels. Individuals whose being is perceived as being primarily 'physical' (or, it might be said, 'animalistic') can be derogated because they remind us of our lowly past, while the geniuses among us can be celebrated as signaling our eventual graduation to the 'higher realm'. As Ritvo wrote, '[c]orollary to this fundamental human/animal dichotomy is the notion that what is good in people reflects their closeness to god (or their divine nature), and what is bad in them reflects their closeness to animals (or their bestial nature)'.[129]

Whatever version the Chain of Being has taken on, moreover, an often unstated presumption of propagandists is that other traits correlate closely with the core values that have been used to order people and groups vertically. Whether 'intelligence', 'religiosity', 'Aryanism', or another value is employed

as the central determination of worth or value, other positive traits are presumed to be found among those at the top of the scale. Critics of eugenics
noted that if the species was bred for intelligence, other positive qualities
(e.g., compassion) might be diminished. Most supporters of eugenic control,
however, simply brushed aside such concerns, noting that, a few exceptions
notwithstanding, controlling for intelligence would raise the overall quality of
the species in other areas as well.

Questioning the full humanity of persons with cognitive disabilities continues
to be a widespread practice, and is often done to sanction calls for their mal-
treatment, medical neglect, or even euthanasia.[130] Peter Singer, perhaps the
most important contemporary ethicist in this field, has questioned whether
mentally disabled humans have a greater claim to moral consideration than
apes, especially if the latter are believed to have 'higher' cognitive abilities. It
is 'speciesist', Singer claims, to treat severely mentally disabled persons with a
higher degree of respect than certain non-human animals – for instance not to
kill them, use them in experiments, or eat them –if the only reason for doing so
is that the former belong to the human species. Just as it is morally inappropriate to treat 'similar' persons of differing races or genders differentially on the
basis of whether they belong to a preferred race or gender, the same principle,
he believes, should be carried over to species membership. In his 'argument
from marginal cases' Singer questions whether we should use severely impaired
persons for experiments instead of chimpanzees and other 'higher' animals.[131]
    The frequent utilization of cognitively disabled persons for experimental
purposes has furthered the view that such individuals have little value to
society and can therefore be treated as guinea pigs. The Fernald radiation and
Willowbrook hepatitis studies, for example, which were described in the previous chapter, were allowed to take place in large part because of the diminished
status accorded to institutionalized persons.[132] Additionally, many of the treatment methodologies which continue to be utilized in response to the persons
who are labeled as mentally retarded also carry with them an implication of
animality. As Wolf Wolfensberger contended, the desire to employ aversive
behavior-modification forms of treatment, such as physical shocks and the use
of restraints, with individuals diagnosed as having cognitive disabilities may
arise in part from the subconscious connection we make between them and
non-human animals.[133]
    The perception of many institutions as 'animalistic' or even death-inducing
environments also continues. Geraldo Rivera, for example, said of the notori-
ous Willowbrook facility in New York that 'virtually every patient in building
Tau was undressed and there was shit everywhere; it looked and smelled like

a poorly kept kennel'.[134] Burton Blatt said of another facility that he was struck by 'the sickening, suffocating smell of feces and urine, decay, dirt and filth, of such strength as to hang in the air and, I thought then and am still not dissuaded, solid enough to be cut or shoveled away'.[135]

Notes

1 Sections of this chapter were originally published in the author's 'Speciesism revisited: The potential for reversibility of the argument from marginal cases (AMC)', *Social Work* 48 (2003), 331–7.

2 B. Shaw, *Man and Superman*, reprint edn. (Baltimore: Penguin Books, 1952), p. 174.

3 H. Von Maltitz, *The Evolution of Hitler's Germany* (New York: McGraw-Hill Book Company, 1973), p. 62. See also Brennan, *Dehumanizing the Vulnerable*, p. 89. Also see P. duBois, *Centaurs and Amazons: Women and the Pre-History of the Great Chain of Being* (Ann Arbor: University of Michigan Press, 1991), p. 13, and Degler, *In Search of Human Nature*, p. 4.

4 J.D. Smith, 'Reflections on mental retardation and eugenics, old and new: Mensa and the Human Genome Project', *Mental Retardation* 32 (1994), 235.

5 Keen, *Faces of the Enemy*, pp. 60–6, 113–16.

6 See, for example, Brennan, *Dehumanizing the Vulnerable*, chapter 11; Keen, *Faces of the Enemy*, pp. 60–2; Levin, *Political Hysteria in America*, p. 6; L. Lowenthal and N. Guterman, *Prophets of Deceit: A Study of Techniques of the American Agitator*, 2nd edn. (Palo Alto, CA: Pacific Books, 1970), pp. 55–8; and Noël, *Intolerance*, pp. 118–19.

7 Keen, *Faces of the Enemy*, p. 61.

8 Blatt, *Exodus from Pandemonium*, p. 161. Another example of a positive animal stereotype in Nazi Germany was Hitler's fascination with the wolf. As Boria Sax noted, the wolf was viewed by Hitler as a fierce predator that had not been weakened through domestication or urbanization. Hitler's nickname was 'the Wolf', which was particularly apropos since the Jews had long been symbolized in Germany as sheep. See B. Sax, *Animals in the Third Reich: Pets, Scapegoats, and the Holocaust* (New York: Continuum International Publishing Group, Inc., 2000), pp. 74–7.

9 George Lakoff and Mark Johnson discuss orientational or spatial metaphors in their book *Metaphors We Live By*, 2nd edn. (Chicago: University of Chicago Press, 2003). As they note, we generally view those items (or persons or groups) that are 'up' as good, and those that are 'down' as bad. It is inherently accepted that on the Chain of Being, as in a sports league or list of academic test scores, the higher one is, the better.

10 P.J. Bowler, *Evolution: The History of an Idea* (Berkeley, CA: University of California Press, 1984), p. 55.

11 A.O. Lovejoy, *The Great Chain of Being* (Cambridge, MA: Harvard University Press, 1966), pp. 193, 198.

12 Quoted in ibid., p. 231.
13 Ibid., p. 184.
14 M.D. Biddiss, *Father of Racist Ideology: The Social and Political Thought of Count Gobineau* (London: Weidenfeld and Nicolson, 1970), p. 119. See also 'Apefooted man', *Eugenics* 1:2 (1928), 27.
15 Lovejoy, *The Great Chain of Being*, p. 234.
16 J.W. Trent, Jr., 'Defectives at the World's Fair: Constructing disability in 1904', *Remedial and Special Education* 19 (1998), 201–11.
17 Dubois, *Centaurs and Amazons*, p. 13.
18 Ibid., p. 12. Also see S.J. Gould, *Ever Since Darwin: Reflections of Natural History* (New York: W.W. Norton and Co., 1981), p. 58.
19 See, for example, Sax, *Animals in the Third Reich*, pp. 50–4; Gasman, *The Scientific Origins of National Socialism*; Gould, *The Mismeasure of Man*, pp. 42, 50; Gould, *The Panda's Thumb* (New York: W.W. Norton and Co., 1980), chapter 16.
20 R. Horsman, *Race and Manifest Destiny: The Origins of American Racial Anglo Saxonism* (Cambridge, MA: Harvard University Press, 1981).
21 C. Lombroso, *Crime: Its Causes and Remedies*, trans. H.P. Horton (Montclair, NJ: Patterson Smith, 1968), p. 367.
22 Ibid., p. 370.
23 Ibid., pp. 52, 365–70.
24 Galton, *Inquiries into Human Faculty and its Development*, p. 43. Also see Deutsch, *Inventing America's 'Worst' Family*, p. 57, and Jackson, *The Borderland of Imbecility*, chapter 5.
25 Cited in M. Tooley, *Abortion and Infanticide* (Oxford: Clarendon Press, 1983), p. 318.
26 See, for example, S.A. Gelb, 'The beast in man: Degeneration and mental retardation, 1900–1920', *Mental Retardation* 33 (1995), 1–9.
27 A.J. Mott, 'The education and custody of the imbecile', in *Proceedings of the National Conference on Charities and Correction* (Boston: Press of Geo. H. Ellis, 1894), p. 168.
28 Quoted in V. Skultans, *Madness and Morals: Ideas on Insanity in the Nineteenth Century* (London: Routledge & Kegan Paul, 1975), p. 249. Also see Jackson, *The Borderland of Imbecility*, p. 137.
29 Ibid., p. 247.
30 Talbot, *Degeneracy*, p. 17; also see pp. 316–17.
31 M. Bancroft, 'Classification of the mentally deficient', in *Proceedings of the National Conference on Charities and Correction* (Boston: Geo. H. Ellis, 1901), p. 196.
32 Talbot, *Degeneracy*, p. 17.
33 See R. Bogdan, 'Exhibiting mentally retarded people for amusement and profit, 1850–1940', *American Journal of Mental Deficiency* 91 (1986), 120–6, and H. Ritvo, 'Border trouble: Shifting the line between people and other animals', *Social Research* 62 (1995), 481–500.

34 Bodgan, 'Exhibiting mentally retarded people', p. 123.
35 Ibid., 125. Also see L. Fielder, *Freaks: Myths and Images of the Secret Self* reprint edn. (New York: Doubleday, 1993), chapter 6.
36 C.F. Goodey, 'The psychopolitics of learning and disability in seventeenth-century thought', in D. Wright and A. Dingby (eds.), *From Idiocy to Mental Deficiency: Historical Perspectives on People with Learning Disabilities* (London: Routledge, 1996), p. 96.
37 Cited in Deutsch, *The Mentally Ill in America*, p. 65. Also see R.C. Scheerenberger, *A History of Mental Retardation* (Baltimore: Paul Brooks Publishing, 1983), p. 95.
38 D. Dix, 'Memorial to the legislature of Massachusetts, 1843', in M. Rosen, G.R. Clark, and M.S. Kivitz (eds.), *The History of Mental Retardation: Collected Papers*, vol. I (Baltimore: University Park Press, 1976), pp. 9–10, 22–3; Foucault, *Madness and Civilization*, pp. 72–5.
39 H. Lane, *The Wild Boy of Aveyron* (New York: Bantam Books, 1976), pp. 53, 64–79.
40 See Trent's *Inventing the Feeble Mind* for an in-depth discussion of the evolving view of the educability of feeble-minded persons in the United States.
41 Pringle, H.N. 'Carnival shows', *Light* 140 (1921), 23.
42 Quoted in L. Thorndike, *A History of Magic and Experimental Science*, vol. VIII, reprint edn. (New York: Columbia University Press, 1964), pp. 471–2.
43 L. Zenderland, *Measuring Minds: Henry Herbert Goddard and the Origins of American Intelligence Testing* (Cambridge: Cambridge University Press, 1998), p. 151.
44 *Eighteenth Biennial Report of the State Home for Feeble-Minded, Winfield, Kansas* (Topeka: Kansas State Printing Plant, 1916), p. 11.
45 See T. R. Robie, 'Towards race betterment', *Birth Control Review* 17:4 (1933), 95.
46 J.H. Kellogg, 'Eugenics Registry Office', in *Proceedings of the First National Conference on Race Betterment* (Battle Creek, MI: Race Betterment Foundation, 1914), p. 565.
47 J.H Kellogg, 'Eugenics and immigration: Needed – a new human race', in *Proceedings of the First National Conference on Race Betterment* (Battle Creek, MI: Race Betterment Foundation, 1914), p. 431.
48 Ibid., pp. 431–2.
49 Guyer, *Being Well-Born*, p. 414.
50 W.G. Lennox, 'Should they live'?, *American Scholar* 7 (1938), 454–5.
51 H.H. Goddard, 'Wanted: A child to adapt', *Survey* 27 (1911), 1004.
52 Black, *War against the Weak*, p. 44. For more on Bell's eugenics, see his 'How to improve the race', *Journal of Heredity* 5:1 (1914), 1–7, R.V. Bruce's *Bell: Alexander Graham Bell and the Conquest of Solitude* (Boston: Little, Brown and Co., 1973), or W.A. Frost, 'A race of human thoroughbreds: An authorized interview with Alexander Graham Bell', *World's Work* 27 (1913), 176–82.
53 W.D. McKim, *Heredity and Human Progress* (New York: G.P. Putnam's Sons, 1901), p. 128.

54 Stern, 'Heredity and environment', p. 188.
55 Whitney, *The Case for Sterilization*, pp. 283–4.
56 .C.B. Davenport, *Heredity in Relation to Eugenics* (New York: Henry Holt and Company, 1911), p. 263 (italics in original).
57 C.B. Davenport, 'The origin and control of mental defectiveness', *Popular Science Monthly* 80 (1912), 90.
58 C.B. Davenport, 'Eugenics and charity', in *Proceedings of the National Conference on Charities and Correction* (Fort Wayne, IN: Fort Wayne Printing Company, 1912), p. 282.
59 Holmes, 'Eugenics', p. 160. For more on the connection between 'reason' and the 'human', see 'Heredity in relation to insanity', Testimony of Representative Kinder, *Congressional Record* (Washington, DC: U.S. Government Printing Office, 12 April 1924), p. 6285, and Lovejoy, *The Great Chain of Being*, pp. 58–9.
60 See, for example, Guyer, 'Sterilization', pp. 52–4; Landman, 'Race betterment by human sterilization', p. 294; Popenoe and Johnson, *Applied Eugenics*, p. 138.
61 A.O. Wright, 'The defective classes', in *Proceedings of the National Conference on Charities and Correction* (Boston: Geo. H. Ellis, 1891), p. 222.
62 See, for example, M.W. Barr, 'Mental defectives and the social welfare,' *Popular Science Monthly* 54 (1899), 749; W.N. Bullard, 'State care of high-grade imbecile girls', in *Proceedings of the National Conference on Charities and Correction* (Press of the Archer Printing Co., 1910), p. 300; Butler, 'A notable factor of social degeneracy', p. 17.
63 G.C. Davenport, 'Hereditary crime', *American Journal of Sociology* 13 (November 1907), 402.
64 H.H. Goddard, 'The basis for state policy: Social investigation and prevention', *Survey* 27 (1912), 1853.
65 C.F. Powlison, 'Behold a sower went forth to sow', *Birth Control Review* 16:1 (1932), 6.
66 Guyer, 'Sterilization', p. 45.
67 See, for example, G.H. Parker, 'The eugenics movement as a public service', *Science* 41 (1915), 347.
68 Zenderland, *Measuring Minds*, p. 198.
69 Goddard, 'The basis for state policy', p. 1854.
70 C.B. Davenport, 'Research in eugenics', *Science* 54 (1921), 394. Also see Davenport's 'Field work an indispensable aid to state care of the socially inadequate', in *Proceedings of the National Conference on Charities and Correction* (Chicago: Hildemann Printing Co., 1915), p. 313.
71 A.C. Rogers, 'Colonizing the feeble-minded', in *Proceedings of the National Conference on Charities and Correction* (Press of Fred J. Heer, 1903), p. 255.
72 H.A. Knox, 'Tests for mental defects', *Journal of Heredity* 5 (1914), 125.
73 Lombroso, *Crime: Its Causes and Remedies*, p. 365.
74 Ibid., p. 52. See also Gould, *Ever Since Darwin*, p. 226.

75 Mott, 'The education and custody of the imbecile', p. 173.
76 Goddard, *The Kallikak Family*, p. 73.
77 Galton, *Inquiries into Human Faculty and its Development*, p. 20.
78 Ibid., p. 20.
79 Kite, 'Unto the third generation', p. 790.
80 Binding and Hoche, 'Permitting the destruction of unworthy life,' p. 263.
81 Pernick, *The Black Stork*, p. 90. The Bollinger baby case of Chicago was the most
    well-known example of the time of refusal to treat a disabled newborn, and led to
    a great deal of discussion related to the ethics of the decision. Pernick's book is
    the best source for the case. Also see 'Doctor to let patient's baby defective die',
    Chicago Tribune (17 November 1915), 1, 'Autopsy puts boy in class of defectives',
    New York Times (18 November 1915), 1, and 'Lets afflicted baby die', *New York
    Times* (28 January 1918), 6. Interestingly, even Helen Keller came out in favor of
    the decision; see J. Gerdtz, 'Disability and euthanasia: The case of Helen Keller
    and the Bollinger baby', *Life and Learning* 16 (2006), 491–500, and her original
    letter supporting the case, H. Keller, 'Physicians' juries for defective babies' (letter
    to the editor), *New Republic* (18 December 1915), 173–4.
82 H.H. Goddard, 'Psychological work among the feeble-minded', *Journal of Psycho
    Asthenics* 12 (1907), 20.
83 Black, *War against the Weak*, p. 52.
84 Mencken, 'Utopia by sterilization', p. 405 (italics in original).
85 Davenport, 'Eugenics and charity', pp. 280–1.
86 Sanger, *The Pivot of Civilization*, p. 93.
87 Stoddard, *Into the Darkness: Nazi Germany Today* (New York: Duell, Sloan &
    Pearce, Inc., 1940), p. 193.
88 Burleigh, *The Third Reich*, p. 360.
89 'Service from imbeciles', *Literary Digest* 53 (1916), 554–5.
90 Stoddard, *The Revolt against Civilization*, p. 89.
91 G.F. Keene, 'The genesis of the defective', in *Proceedings of the National Conference
    on Charities and Correction* (Press of Fred J. Heer, 1904), p. 413.
92 Pernick, *The Black Stork*, p. 49. See also Zenderland, *Measuring Minds*, p. 148.
93 Quoted in W.H. Tucker, *The Science and Politics of Racial Research* (Urbana:
    University of Illinois Press, 1996), p. 62.
94 Davenport, *Heredity in Relation to Eugenics*, p. 262.
95 W.J. Hickson, 'The criminal in everyday life', in *Proceedings of the Third National
    Conference on Race Betterment* (Battle Creek, MI: Race Betterment Foundation,
    1928), p. 148.
96 Davenport, 'The origin and control of mental defectiveness', p. 89. See also his
    Heredity in Relation to Eugenics, p. 262.
97 See A.E. Wiggam, *The New Decalogue of Science* (Indianapolis: Bobbs-Merrill
    Company, 1923), p. 102; Kellogg, 'Eugenics and immigration', p. 433.
98 'Intelligence wane seen by Dr. Hooton', *New York Times* (18 February 1937), 1.
99 'Hooton finds man reverting to ape', *New York Times* (4 December 1937), 27.

See also '"Saving Homo sapiens": Professor Hooton sees hope only in applying eugenics', *New York Times* (28 February 1927), section XII, 8.

100 See, for example, Lennox, 'Should they live?', p. 457; 'Mercy death law ready for Albany', *New York Times* (14 February 1939), 2; H.S. Jennings, 'Health progress and race progress: Are they compatible?', in *American Association for the Study of the Feebleminded: Proceedings and Addresses of the Fifty-First Annual Session* (American Association for the Study of the Feebleminded, 1927), p. 234; McKim, *Heredity and Human Progress*, pp. 128–9; Baldwin, 'The psychology of mental deficiency', p. 84; Pernick, *The Black Stork*, p. 95; Kirkbride, 'The army of sorrow', p. 228; E.A. Irwin, 'Fragments of humanity', *The Survey* (2 March 1912), 1875; A. Lyons, 'Ungraded parents', *Education* 38 (1917), 338; Ward, 'The crisis in our immigration policy', p. 39; Binding and Hoche, 'Permitting the destruction of unworthy life', p. 261; 'Burned-out human husks' quotation from in F. Wertham, *A Sign for Cain: An Exploration of Human Violence* (New York: Macmillan Co., 1966), p. 189; Whitney, *The Case for Sterilization*, p. 284.

101 H. Olson, 'The menace of the half-man', in *Proceedings of the Third Race Betterment Conference* (Battle Creek, MI: Race Betterment Foundation, 1928), pp. 122–47.

102 G.H. Knight, 'Prevention from a legal and moral standpoint', in *Proceedings of the National Conference on Charities and Correction* (Boston: Geo. H. Ellis, 1898), p. 306.

103 'Was the doctor right? Some independent opinions', *Independent*, 85:3500 (1916), 23.

104 A.H. Estabrook, 'The Tribe of Ishmael', in *Eugenics, Genetics and the Family*, vol. I: *Scientific Papers of the Second International Congress of Eugenics* (Baltimore: Williams & Wilkins Company, 1923), p. 400.

105 Stern, 'Heredity and environment', p. 180.

106 Kite, 'The "Piney's"', p. 40. The term 'Piney' came from the region of New Jersey where Kite spent much of her time, and was perhaps an early pseudonym for the Kallikak family, who inhabited the Pine Barrens.

107 Butler, 'A notable factor of social degeneracy', p. 19.

108 Rafter, *White Trash*, p. 26.

109 Ibid., p. 27.

110 Ibid., p. 26.

111 A.H. Estabrook, 'A two-family apartment', *Survey* 29 (1913), 853–4. Also see Mina Sessions, 'Feeble-minded in Ohio', *Journal of Heredity* 8 (1917), 291–7. Also see Nies, *Eugenic Fantasies*, p. 35.

112 Kostir, *The Family of Sam Sixty*, p. 29.

113 Stoddard, *The Revolt against Civilization*, pp. 233, 238.

114 Hadden, *The Science of Eugenics and Sex Life*, p. 3.

115 C.B. Davenport, 'Importance of heredity to the state', *Indiana Bulletin* (September 1913), 402–4.

116 F. Kennedy, 'Euthanasia: To be or not to be', *Colliers* 103 (20 May 1939), 15. For

more on the major American supporters of eugenic euthanasia, see M.L. Offen, 'Dealing with "defectives": Foster Kennedy and William Lennox on eugenics', *Neurology* 61 (2003), 668–73.

117 Lennox, 'Should they live?', p. 457.

118 M. Shipley, 'The sterilization of defectives', *American Mercury* 15 (1928), 454.

119 Binding and Hoche, 'Permitting the destruction of unworthy life', p. 263.

120 Quoted in R.J. Lifton, *The Nazi Doctors: Medical Killing and the sychology of Genocide* (New York: Basic Books, Inc., 1986), p. 62.

121 Burleigh, *Death and Deliverance*, p. 194; see also pp. 184–93.

122 Burleigh, *The Third Reich: A New History*, p. 379.

123 See Albert Deutsch, *The Shame of the States*, reprint edn. (New York: Arno Press, 1973), chapter 10, on 'Euthanasia through neglect'.

124 Pernick, *The Black Stork*, p. 10. Also see Black, *War against the Weak*, pp. 254–6.

125 M.A. Elks, 'The "lethal chamber": Further evidence for the euthanasia option', *Mental Retardation* 31 (1993), 205.

126 Ibid., 201.

127 Sax, *Animals in the Third Reich*, chapter 11.

128 Gould, *The Mismeasure of Man*, chapter 5.

129 Ritvo, 'Border trouble', p. 482.

130 O'Brien, 'Speciesism revisited'. Also see J. Fletcher, *The Ethics of Genetic Control* (Garden City, NY: Anchor Books, 1974), pp. 170–1.

131 P. Singer, 'All animals are equal', in T. Regan and P. Singer (eds.), *Animal Rights and Human Obligations*, reprint edn. (Englewood Cliffs, NJ: Prentice Hall, 1989), and *Animal Liberation: A New Ethics for Our Treatment of Animals* (New York: Avon Books, 1975), pp. 16–20. For additional information on speciesism and the argument from marginal cases, see D.A. Dombrowski, *Babies and Beasts: The Argument from Marginal Cases* (Urbana: University of Illinois Press, 1997), and O'Brien, 'Speciesism revisited'.

132 Primary sources noted Chapter 2 n. 112 above. Also see H.K. Beecher, *Research and the Individual* (Boston: Little, Brown and Co, 1970), pp. 122–7.

133 Wolfensberger, *The Principle of Normalization in Human Services*, p. 19.

134 G. Rivera, *Willowbrook* (New York: Random House, 1972), p. 78.

135 Blatt, *Exodus from Pandomonium*, pp. 13–14.

4

THE WAR AND NATURAL
CATASTROPHE METAPHORS:
THE MORON AS AN ENEMY FORCE

Congenitally incapable of adjusting themselves to an advanced social order, the degenerate inevitably become its enemies – particularly those 'high-grade defectives' who are the natural fomenters of social unrest.[1]

'Undesirable' community groups, especially those which can be framed as potentially destructive to society at large, are often described through the employment of military or natural catastrophe metaphors. In such cases, the group is put forth as a primary and imminent threat to society. Taking action against the group can thereupon be put forth as a matter of self-preservation, and failing to support such community protection measures is similarly described as a sign of mushy sentimentality, cowardice, disloyalty, or even outright treachery. If a problem can be framed as a 'war', the public may feel compelled to accept sacrifices in order to fight it. These sacrifices may be economic or social, and may include, for example, a substantial financial outlay, usually from taxes, or a diminishment of civil liberties for certain groups – or for the population as a whole – in the name of national security. Social control policies that are in keeping with the war or natural catastrophe metaphor include such measures as deportation, imprisonment, closely monitoring the movement and actions of target group members, and restricting their entrance into the country or their freedom of assembly or speech.

The war metaphor is often invoked to bring a particular issue or target group to the forefront of public attention as the principal threat to the nation or the major cause that needs to be addressed by policymakers. At any one time, a rather large array of social problems and potential target groups are available for public consideration and various policy responses. In the United States currently, for example, we must consider policies related to such diverse sociopolitical issues as foreign and domestic terrorism, long-term solvency of the social security and health care systems, same-sex marriage, economic stability, and child sexual abuse. A large community of interest that includes producers, investors, professional service providers, politicians, media representatives, advocacy groups, and other assorted stakeholders has coalesced around each of these issues. These groups compete with one another for public exposure, funding, and an expansion of the sphere of influence within which they can operate. Importantly, those social problems that are successfully framed and accepted by the public as domestic 'wars' are likely to receive an extensive degree of financial and other forms of support, since waging a war against a social problem or presumably threatening community subgroup does not lend itself to a half-hearted response.

War or military metaphors are obviously a natural means of framing the opposition group when it is viewed as engaging in a conspiracy against the nation, or thought to be planning some form of attack, as in the fight against communism or terrorism. However, even when the fear that is engendered against such groups is based partly on factual information, alarm movements may gain a great deal of impetus from pre-existing hatreds, the exploitation of traumatic events, the egotism and ambition of some of the most voracious supporters of control measures, the resources provided by entrenched bureaucratic and corporate institutions that profit from the fear, and the media's proliferation of social myths related to the group in question.

As with Japanese internment, the threat that the group is said to present may become so considerable that control policies are extended to persons who have associated with those targeted or even to individuals who simply belong to a specific ethnic or religious group or are of the same nationality as actual or alleged perpetrators. The burden of proof moves from accuser to the accused during the time of war, and the precept that one is 'innocent until proven guilty' and other aspects of due process may be presented as the luxuries of a more peaceful era that cannot be afforded during the current troubled times. Advocates of control often argue that it is better to err on the side of restricting the rights of innocent persons who may belong to the opposition than on the side of placing innocent citizens in harm's way. The former is presented as merely inconvenient, the latter as potentially devastating and a sign of national weakness.

Through the war metaphor the propagandist positions herself or himself as a protector of the nation, or a vigilant and prescient visionary who can see a looming disaster long before others. As with the organism metaphor, proactive measures are said to be necessary for protecting the nation. Waiting for a potential enemy to strike prior to taking action is presented as similar to allowing a plague to establish itself before instituting public health measures.

Importantly, the opposition is depicted not only as sneaky and secretive but, as noted in the previous chapter, as not fighting fairly. The two primary advantages that can take it to victory are public indifference of the threat it poses and a dishonorable means of engagement.

During an alarm period, members of the target group are frequently accused of attempting to 'pass' as non-stigmatized members of the community. For example, many Jewish-owned businesses in the late 1800s and early 1900s were operated under non-Jewish names, or by proprietors who changed their names.[2] During the 1910s and 1920s many Japanese in California operated farms under the names of others, since they were forbidden by law to own their own property.[3] In each case there was a viable rationale for the action: the former was precipitated in part by widespread discrimination against Jewish-operated businesses, and the latter by state policies that kept Japanese from owning property. Those who call for a restriction of rights from group members, however, are likely to point to such subterfuge as emblematic of the group's efforts to gain power or wealth covertly. Especially if the group can be perceived as having a foreign 'allegiance' or values that are supposedly contrary to 'American' ones, members can also readily be accused as being potentially treasonous.

The struggle against the target class is therefore presented as a matter of self- defense. Propagandists and advocates of control position themselves not as heartless mean-spirited bullies but rather as defenders of hearth and home. As Sam Keen noted in his book *Faces of the Enemy*, war posters and other forms of propaganda frequently include visual images or descriptions of women and children who have been or will be harmed by the enemy.[4] As a result, the masculinity of males who want to study the issue further or investigate the actual degree of danger that exists can be called into question. Even the brutality of the Nazis was supported within Germany as the only way of defending the nation against Jewish aggression. As Cohn wrote, for example, a principal theme of anti-Jewish publications such as *Der Sturmer* was that of Jews engaging in the ritual murder of German children and raping young Aryan girls.[5]

Another important characteristic of alarm periods is that the fight against the target group is presented as a zero-sum game, lacking any possibility of compromise and thus any reason for negotiation with the 'enemy'. Since the opposition cannot be trusted, negotiation would be fruitless and would only buy the enemy time to further organize and conspire. In some cases, moreover, the characteristics of the group that are most threatening are said to be inherent and non-malleable (e.g., the fecundity of 'undesirable' immigrant groups, the greediness of Jews, the untruthfulness of communists, the brutality and hyper-sexuality of African-Americans), and therefore any possibility of compromise that involves their mitigating these behaviors is said to be unattainable anyway.

The perception that the target group has the potential to devastate the nation in a similar fashion to a natural catastrophe is closely related to the war metaphor. The group may be described, for example, as a 'flood', 'tsunami', 'avalanche', or 'tornado'. In cases where a group has not engaged in any harmful activities, but presumably is involved in the planning of such, it may even be depicted as a dormant volcano that may erupt at any time. In most cases, however, a principal difference between the war metaphor and the natural catastrophe metaphor relates to the motives of the target group. Within the context of the former, the harm it poses is normally intentional and motivated by malice or greed. As with a 'flood' of immigrants, however, those described by natural catastrophe metaphors may not even be aware of the damage they are alleged to be inflicting on the nation. As this chapter describes, however, this standard does not always apply. While morons were generally framed as unknowingly posing a threat to the nation, the military metaphor was still a fairly prevalent mode of describing the 'war on feeble-mindedness'.

Finally, it should be noted that either the war or the natural catastrophe metaphor is especially likely to be employed if the target group is large and imposing, and particularly if the group is framed as a rapidly growing threat, through extensive immigration, rapid procreation, the ability to dupe 'weak-minded' or 'wrong-thinking' citizens to aid in their cause, or fears of miscegenation that result in a crisis of identity within the population.

A grave and imminent crisis: the 'war' on moronity

Just as many eugenicists contended that the 'submerged tenth' of the population was a spreading cancer threatening to infect healthy portions of the social body or a collection of animalistic entities that did not deserve the full range of human rights, it was also described as an enemy force with the potential to destroy the nation. Rhetoric that expressed the nature of the imminent crisis caused by an expanding body of morons within the country often took on an unmistakable urgency: a plea for the very survival of 'civilized' culture. Eugenicists argued that not only was the United States no longer moving forward as a people, but the race was actually beginning to degenerate because of the expansion of the moron population through massive immigration and the remarkable fecundity among the lower (and presumably less intelligent) classes. In contrast with the situation in Nazi Germany, where positive and negative eugenics were equally supported, eugenics in the United States was almost exclusively justified not as a method of directing the evolution of the

species upward, but rather as a means of mitigating continued 'race deterioration'. The movement was driven not by hope but by fear.

The need for military readiness seemed to support concerns about the
intellectual (and thus physical) weakness of the country's population. Shortly
after the entrance of the United States entrance into World War I, a group of
psychologists, many of whom supported eugenic policies, developed an intelligence test which recruits were required to take. This test allowed the army to
place soldiers in the military position for which they appeared best suited. The
most astonishing finding of these tests was that they seemed to demonstrate
that the average mentality of adult males in the nation bordered on feeble-
mindedness.[6] The results were especially disconcerting, one eugenicist wrote,
because 'the obviously feeble-minded ... had already been weeded out before
the tests were made'.[7] The test results were presented by Carl Brigham in the
1923 book *A Study of American Intelligence*, and specifically provided evidence
for the limited intellectual capacity of recent immigrants from southern and
eastern European nations, as comparisons of test scores had been made on the
basis of the recruits' nationalities.[8]

Eugenicists clearly viewed the feeble-minded and other degenerates as a
portion of the populace that was situated in an antagonistic position in relation to the rest of the community. Articles with titles such as 'The imbecile and
epileptic *versus* the tax-payer and the community' and 'The case of the nation
vs. the feebleminded' supported the prevailing belief that morons were an
internal enemy force whose restriction and control needed to be addressed.[9]
This enemy force, moreover, could presumably bring the country to its knees
if not controlled through restrictive social policies. Under a diagram of the
Kallikak family, Albert Wiggam referred to the 'bad' Kallikaks as 'nation-
destroying descendants',[10] and Michael Guyer, writing about 'degenerate'
immigrants, stated that since 'we must inevitably mingle our life blood with
that of such invading hordes, or possibly be replaced by them, our very existence as a nation is at stake'.[11] Others wrote that degeneracy 'not only handi-
caps society but threatens its very existence',[12] that 'drastic action' to control
the procreation of the feeble-minded was the only way to 'avert grave disaster
from the nation',[13] and that feeble-mindedness was 'one of the most terrible
forces acting against society'.[14] Speaking of those morons who remained 'at-
large' in the community, J.M. Murdoch, the superintendent of a Pennsylvania
institution, said that protecting the nation from external enemies would be
largely ineffective if 'a known and insidious danger in our midst' was not
likewise controlled.[15] In keeping with the eugenical framing of feeble-minded
women as especially dangerous to the community, Alexander Johnson, who
was attached to the training school at Vincland, New Jersey wrote that women

'constitute a graver danger to the prosperity of the state than a foreign war or native pestilence'.[16]

Eugenicists employed the most compelling language possible in an effort to describe the extent of the moron threat.[17] One physician said that the 'wave of degeneracy' sweeping the land was 'so appalling in its magnitude that it staggers the mind and threatens to destroy the republic; numbering more victims than have been claimed in all of the wars and all of the epidemics of acute diseases that have swept the country within 200 years'.[18] Still others contended that morons were 'monstrous, indescribable things which a Hercules with a thousand lives could not vanquish in untold generations',[19] and that the 'menace of low mentality is perhaps the greatest danger that confronts any nation or civilization'.[20] The menace of the feeble-minded was also said to be the 'most acute crisis' in the history of the race,[21] and eugenics was thus the 'paramount duty of the hour' and a 'truism not to be questioned'.[22] Eugenicists stressed that the extent of the threat was so grave that control of defectiveness was not just one of a number of social reforms that would improve society. It was, indeed, the lynchpin of social reform. Since feeble-mindedness presumably caused most other social problems, including poverty, alcoholism, child neglect, and immorality, any progress in dealing with these other problems required some degree of differential population control. Eugenic policies, supporters contended, provided an underpinning for all of the 'euthenic' efforts that would define Progressivism.

Some directly infused their recommendations for eugenic control with military rhetoric. Harry Haiselden, the leading American advocate of euthanasia during the eugenic era, supported this drastic measure because, as he wrote, 'we have been invaded', and our 'streets are infested with an Army of the Unfit – a dangerous, vicious army of death and dread'. This army was, Haiselden said, composed of 'horrid things that drag themselves through our streets by day and night'.[23] Similarly, Martin Barr wrote that feeble-mindedness 'is an enemy that attacks not our frontiers but our hearthstones', and that '[w]e have reached the point where we must conquer it, lest it should conquer us'.[24] To Henry Goddard the feeble-minded segment of the population constituted an 'army of more than five hundred thousand persons [that] furnishes the recruits for the ranks of the criminals, the paupers, the prostitutes ... and others of our social misfits'.[25] Lastly, Caroline Robinson wrote that among 'our 30 million dependents there are some – maybe one million, maybe ten, against whose continuation it is time to move. It is our responsibility to cut off a bit of the degenerate tail-end of this menacing army, whether the degenerated tail turns out to be a furlong of the army or a mile of it, and even if we can only clip a yard off for the present.'[26]

As mentioned above, a central belief of the immigration restriction movement was that the huge number of southern and eastern European immigrants
who were coming from overseas constituted an undesirable foreign incur-
sion into the United States not unlike a wartime invasion.[27] One writer, for
example, noted that the invasion of the United States through immigration
was 'equal to one hundred and fifty full regiments of one thousand each'.[28] As
feeble-mindedness came to be more closely associated with the 'new immigration', the moron threat was greatly enhanced by the invasion rhetoric that had
long framed the immigration restriction debate. In his book *The Sieve*, Weiss
discussed several cases of deportable immigrants, including some who were
not allowed to enter the country and others who slipped by. In discussing
one of the latter cases, involving a Russian woman with an 'idiotic' child, he
wondered what became of them, and speculated that the boy might 'produce
a whole regiment of idiots, drunkards, lunatics, public charges, in the next fifty
years, who would cost the state thousands of dollars to support, later on'.[29]
According to Harry Laughlin, from a eugenic standpoint 'military conquest by
a superior people would be highly preferable to a conquest by immigration' of
an inferior group.[30]

Eugenics and the curtailment of civil liberties

Advocates of eugenics realized that in order to garner public support for their
cause they would have to show valid rationales for infringing on individual
liberties. The danger that morons and other defectives posed to the rest of the
community, they argued, justified their control. George Knight, a physician
and institutional superintendent, in discussing an early proposal that feeble-
minded persons be made wards of the state so that they could be forcibly
committed, wrote in 1898: 'I am well aware that this suggestion carried out
would strike a blow directly at the root of what is called the law of individual
right, but I claim that the mentally unfit have no individual right to reproduce
themselves.'[31] When the rights of one group of persons, Barr added, conflicted
with the rights of others, some form of governmental control was warranted.[32]
Noting that sterilizations and institutionalizations were increasing in the
1930s, even as the 'menace of the feeble-minded' was waning, Wendy Kline
wrote that many were sympathetic to the argument that '[i]n a time of crisis,
personal rights had to be sacrificed for the common good', and stated that the
economic collapse during the Great Depression provided a receptive environment for the diminution of certain rights.[33]

As noted in Chapter 2, one method by which civil liberties are frequently
restricted when a group presumably poses a threat to the nation is to require

members of the group to identify themselves (or be identified by others), formally register with a bureaucratic authority, and, in many cases, 'carry papers'. One of Davenport's goals was to make the Eugenics Record Office a central storehouse for such records. He, along with other supporters, believed that so long as people added to the larger pool of genetic traits through children and later ancestors, their family traits constituted a matter of public interest.

Adolf Hitler realized the importance of implementing social control measures in a time of crisis. He knew that the wide-scale implementation of the sterilization law would be more acceptable in Germany during the early 1930s than at any other time because of the country's own economic problems. The impact of the worldwide depression was profound in Germany, in part because the nation was already experiencing financial troubles resulting from World War I reparations. Hitler also realized that the 'euthanasia' program would encounter less resistance if it was not initiated until Germany was at war. The conflict would not only relegate the killings to the 'back pages' of public discussion, but additionally would add to the argument that even this degree of restriction might be necessary in view of the circumstances. Thus he waited until the 1939 invasion of Poland to begin the T-4 euthanasia program.[34] 'The association of euthanasia and war', Proctor noted, 'was not fortuitous. If the healthy could sacrifice their lives in time of war, then why should the sick not do the same?'[35] Because of the importance of the metaphorical comparison between morons and soldiers within the context of eugenic rhetoric, the topic deserves an extended discussion.

Soldiers and traitors: parenthood during the eugenic era

As noted above, in their rationales for both positive and negative eugenic programs, eugenic writings frequently alluded to soldiers and military service as a relevant point of contrast with the moron. Many of those in the American movement, foreshadowing the later arguments of some of their German counterparts, compared parenthood to soldiering, noting that the two were equally important for ensuring the continued strength of the nation. An underlying theme in the advocacy of eugenics was that without 'fit' parents, there would be no soldiers. In a 1924 article in the *Journal of Heredity*, Ernest Dodge addressed these potential parents:

> Where two parents such as you ... shall unite to form a home, there must emerge *more than two* children to form an increased part of the coming world. This is your assigned and positive duty to society, your soldierhood to the great human commonwealth. You will not even desire to be slackers in this warfare against the insidious forces which would thwart the divine purposes of evolution.[36]

Such parents, he added, cannot shirk their duty to society, but 'must come to recognize that they are drafted for world service by a draft board higher than any established by man'.[37] Theodore Roosevelt too, who had strong concerns about the potential for 'race suicide', compared potential 'fit' parents to conscripts, and said that the former should not 'shirk their duty' to the nation.[38] In *Being Well-Born*, Michael Guyer asked whether 'the able-bodied and able-minded men and women who refuse to marry and rear children fit to carry on civilization [are] as much shirkers in their duty to their nation as the coward who slinks away from the dangers of war.'[39] According to Charles Davenport, by bearing 'fit' children for the nation, young women 'do the work that none others can do and which is a patriotic service no less sublime than that rendered on the fields of battle'.[40]

While American and German eugenicists, for the most part, had a collegial relationship during the early 1930s, tensions arose as war clouds loomed and it became obvious that Germany was surpassing the United States in the implementation of eugenic policies. The control of human breeding fused with the preparedness for military conflict as eugenicists warned that those nations that were best able to control the constitution of their populace would have a definite advantage in future wars as well as in other forms of international competition (e.g., economic development, technological innovation). This was especially relevant since the interval between the beginnings of the two world wars, about twenty-four years, was approximately the amount of time it would have taken one side to 're-supply' its fighting force through a strong positive eugenic program. Several decades before World War II Harry Haiselden alluded to the connection between eugenics and national strength when attempting to support his decision to allow the Bollinger baby to die: 'there are no defectives among the Japanese. The surgeons of Nippon often fail to tie the umbilical cord. As a result, the Japanese are a wonderfully vigorous race deservedly coming into world prominence.'[41]

Members of the American movement, such as Clarence Campbell, the President of the Eugenics Research Association, not only were envious of Germany's rapid progress in population control, but also worried that their own country was falling behind. Campbell called on Americans not only to consider 'racial' and eugenic aspects when marrying, but to increase their child-bearing. 'Patriotism', he said, 'carries with it a willingness on the part of individuals not only to cooperate in the common interest but to sacrifice individualistic aims and submit themselves to discipline in the ultimate interest of the group'.[42] Similarly, Robert Proctor wrote that as 'early as 1931 the Nazis introduced into parliament legislation requiring that "anyone who attempts to curb artificially the natural fertility of the German people" be punished by imprisonment for "racial treason"'.[43]

As one might assume, eugenicists held that if 'fit' parents had a patriotic duty to reproduce, their 'unfit' peers had a similar duty to the nation to refrain from breeding. As discussed above, comparisons between feeble-minded persons and soldiers served to provide a stark contrast between what were taken to be the most valuable and most valueless lives. Eugenicists argued that while the former were weak and dependent, and did little to aid society, the latter were strong, essential members of a vibrant community who were willing to make the ultimate sacrifice for the good of the nation. Because 'the public welfare' periodically called upon its 'best citizens' to give up their lives for their country in wartime, Oliver Wendell Holmes wrote in the *Buck v. Bell* decision, it could also call upon the feeble-minded segment of the community to make a lesser sacrifice by becoming sterile.[44] According to Mary Dudziak, the 'allusion to wartime deaths' would naturally lead those who read the *Buck* decision, many of whose family members had fought or died in World War I, to 'agree that the nation's wars had taken the lives of those who were more worthy of citizenship than the likes of Carrie Buck'.[45]

One of the more creative recommendations for a program of negative eugenics was that 'mentally deficient' persons actually be enlisted to fight the nation's wars. A physician from Harvard Medical School proposed, at a 1917 meeting of the American Association for the Study of the Feeble-Minded, that morons be placed on the front lines during World War I as a way of both adding to the fighting force and ensuring the demise of such persons:

> One more question along the line of the particular consideration of this problem. It has been suggested that this type of individual [morons] should be excluded from the militia. I think there are two sides of this problem, and that an entirely opposite suggestion might well be entertained. I should like to know what the experts, from whom we have heard, would think about this as a possible way of ridding the state of this overwhelming number of individuals. I should not propose that they be put into the army without diagnosis, or without proper supervision there, but it seems to me that as a means of sweeping them off the earth it would be a very good one.[46]

Imperiled democracy and eugenic control

Many eugenicists were quick to point out that the threat of the growing 'defective' population was heightened by concerns that these people would hijack the democratic process itself, thereupon passing social reform measures that would ensure the exacerbation of race suicide. Drawing on earlier arguments by the British population theorist Thomas Malthus, social Darwinistic eugenicists decried the fact that in a republic, politicians would cater to the needs of the masses.[47] As rights and privileges were given to those who did not 'deserve' them, in order to garner votes, individual initiative would presumably diminish. If the electorate was composed increasingly of feeble-minded individuals, the argument continued, policies that benefitted them, such as economic entitlements, would be embraced by politicians who needed their support. As taxation increased as a result of these policies, the more 'fit' segments of the population would thereupon constrain their procreative output, in large measure because high taxation would limit their ability to provide the economic support necessary for their own children. A 1932 article in the *Journal of Heredity* held that

> whereas the multiplication of the less capable – and even the definitely unfit – is encouraged by subsidies, the more capable minority are hindered from rearing even moderate families by the drastic taxation which is necessary to provide those subsidies ... We must assume that the present political system, with its subsidies to the inferior at the expense of the superior, will continue unless its economic and biological unsoundness manifests itself in some national catastrophe.[48]

Michael Guyer expressed frustration at the fact that 'in a democracy the vote of each of these [morons] has just as much weight as that of the most enlightened citizen',[49] and Lothrop Stoddard stated that 'democracy was never intended for degenerates, and a nation breeding freely of the sort that must continually be repressed is not headed toward an extension of democratic liberties'.[50] Seth Humphrey warned readers that if a large number of 'incompetents' were allowed to vote, the result would be disastrous. He recommended, therefore, that an intelligence test be given to all prospective voters to ensure that only 'competent citizens' could vote.[51] Earnest Hooton urged eugenic control as a necessary precursor for maintaining a sound system of government. Paraphrasing Abraham Lincoln, he wrote that 'we must either do some biological house-cleaning or delude ourselves with the futile hope that a government of the unfit, for the unfit, and by the unfit will not perish from the earth'.[52]

Concerns regarding the ability of persons with limited mentality being able to vote came about at the time when other related threats to democracy were voiced. From anarchists, socialists, and communists gaining political power to labor activism and its impact on the polls and to the rising strength, especially in large cities such as New York and Boston, of Jewish, Irish, and other 'outsider' immigrant or ethnic groups gaining power, the early decades of the century were marked by fears that democracy would fall into the wrong hands. From the standpoint of many eugenicists, feeble-minded persons were the perfect 'dupes' for any of these groups, ready to sell their votes to any and all comers regardless of the possible consequences.

Internal enemies of the state: the moron as criminal

The status of the feeble-minded as an internal archenemy of the people was greatly fostered by the perception that they were responsible for a large portion of the criminal behavior that took place within society.[53] 'After the conclusions of [the Italian criminologist Cesare] Lombroso on criminal anthropology had come to be more or less discredited', wrote S.J. Holmes, 'the distinguishing feature of criminals was sought rather in their low intelligence than their physical peculiarities'.[54] Goddard contended that '[t]he best material out of which to make criminals ... is feeble-mindedness',[55] and, to Walter Fernald, '[e]very imbecile, especially the high-grade imbecile, is a potential criminal, needing only the proper environment and opportunity for the development and expression of his criminal tendencies'.[56] Studies conducted at the time purported to show that a very large percentage of the prison population was feeble-minded, and these criminals were frequently presented as incapable of rehabilitation, since their problems lay in their defective brains.[57]

In *The Family of Sam Sixty*, one of the eugenic family studies, Mary Koster noted that while morons frequently engaged in criminal activities, the crimes they committed were not illegal acts that required ingenuity or complex planning. They were normally acts of violence that arose from a 'lack of self control'.[58] Morons were said to be principally responsible for a large variety of crimes, including arsons, automobile accidents, and even homicides.[59] Johnstone wrote that '[m]any deaths are to be laid at the doors of the degenerates',[60] and the *Buck* decision held that 'instead of waiting to execute degenerate offspring for crime', we should 'prevent those who are manifestly unfit from continuing their kind'.[61] Clairette Armstrong went so far as to suggest that if nations would limit the birth of those with low intelligence, 'even wars ... would be greatly diminished'.[62]

Criminalistic terminology can be found throughout the writings of the eugenicists. Institutionalized feeble-minded persons were often referred to as 'inmates', discharge from such facilities was termed 'parole', these discharged clients remained on 'permanent probation', and those persons presumed to be morons who were not in facilities were said to be 'at large' in the community.[63] The 'defective delinquent' or 'moral imbecile' was another staple of the alarm period. These terms described those individuals, not necessarily but often diagnosed as feeble-minded, who had a propensity to commit crimes, usually because of a lack of willpower or knowledge of right and wrong. Such persons, it was said, had a callous indifference to the suffering they caused, and were incapable of improvement.[64]

Many eugenicists argued that, because of the criminal propensity of the moron, mandatory segregation was the only way to relieve the community of the problem. Even sterilization, while it would ensure that the individual's 'genetic defects' would not be passed on, failed to protect society from the criminal behavior in which feeble-minded persons might engage. Institutional confinement was considered 'the only means of protecting the public, not only from the moral menace of the feebleminded, but also from the danger of murderous assault, arson and crimes of sexual perversion'.[65] One of the foremost advocates of preventive criminology, Chicago's Harry Olsen, contended that the court system could almost be eliminated if 'defectives' were recognized before they committed crimes and removed to 'farm colonies'.[66] 'Good psychiatrists', he felt, 'can identify them when they are babies.' He added that to allow such persons to have '"one chance", and thus to start them on the treadmill of crime and restraint, is no kindness to them'.[67] Walter Fernald recommended that prison inmates should be tested for feeble-mindedness, and that those so labeled should be 'transferred to permanent custody' in an institution once their sentences had expired.[68]

The birth differential and the threat of racial ruination

The fear that was directed at persons who were diagnosed as feeble-minded during the eugenic era was fostered in large part by the birth differential argument, which greatly exacerbated concerns about the spread of degenerate conditions through the rest of society. As noted previously, many eugenicists contended that differential birth rates were caused in large part by social welfare and economic reforms as well as by sanitation and disease control initiatives. While seeing them as beneficial in supporting persons in need, many believed that these social reform measures served to foster the survival and propagation of the 'unfit', thus having a dysgenic impact on society.[69]

The birth differential argument could easily fit within any of the conceptual metaphors discussed in this book. Within the organism metaphor, a rapidly reproducing destructive subgroup can be easily viewed as a cancer or bacillus. Within the animal metaphor, rabbits, roaches, or any other highly fecund species have often fostered the same image. The immorality and lack of control that lead to such wanton reproduction is related to the religious metaphor, and the depersonalization and focus on the mass of the group that often arise with the birth differential argument are part and parcel of the object metaphor.

An extended discussion of the argument is included here, however, since it probably relates more to the war metaphor than to any other. The birth differential argument played a very important role in fostering the belief that the menace of the feeble-minded was not just one of many social problems to be addressed through reform measures, but the crucial problem of the time. A distinguishing feature of the war metaphor as it was employed within eugenic writings was the immediacy and intensity with which the spread of moronity needed to be fought. There was no time to waste, nor to gather additional research on the issue, because these persons were increasing at such an astonishing pace.

Moreover, propagandists noted that the problem needed to be fought on two fronts, since moronity was increasing not only through dysgenic reproduction within the country, but also through the immigration of feeble-minded persons and other 'defectives'. Additionally, birth differential fears fit well here because of their actuarial nature. Just as numbers (of soldiers on each side, weaponry, allies, economic support, etc.) are important in a war, and tell much about the nature of the struggle, so too the menace of the feeble-minded was stoked by numbers, with the enemy being seen as an imposing, expanding, potentially overwhelming horde of morons and other defectives.

A seminal feature of many alarm periods, the birth differential argument was strongly influenced by Malthus's writings on population growth, which predated the eugenic era by a full century.[70] Another important early influence was General F.A. Walker, who was Superintendent of the Census in the United States in 1870 and 1880. Walker expressed grave concerns about the expansion of the 'new' immigrant population (e.g., Irish, Italians) in relation to the population of Anglo-Americans during this period. He contended that even though millions of immigrants were entering the country during these decades, the nation's overall population was not increasing much. His explanation for this was that the 'native' population was restricting its own rate of growth, in large part because of fears that its children would not fare well in direct labor competition with the children of these immigrants. It was not, Walker argued, that 'American' children did not have the skills or abilities to compete with foreigners, but rather that they were more civilized, and could not live in the substandard conditions that immigrants endured. The latter, therefore, could perform the same jobs at lower wages.[71] Those who warned of eugenic or racial deterioration frequently invoked Walker's research. In *The Rising Tide of Color*, for example, Lothrop Stoddard quoted Prescott Hall, one of the leaders of the immigration restriction movement, as saying that 'immigration to any country of a given stratum of population tends to sterilize all strata of higher social and economic levels already in that country'.[72]

Walker's arguments bolstered the fears of race suicide that took hold during the early decades of the twentieth century, and were exacerbated by the growing interest in birth control among the upper and middle classes. Statistical demographics pertaining to the relative numbers of children in immigrant and 'native' families seemed to provide evidence substantiating these concerns.[73] Harry Laughlin, for example, contended that if reproduction rates remained unchanged, the descendants of new immigrants would be a majority of the population within four generations.[74]

Shortly after the turn of the century, the birth differential fears that characterized xenophobia came to be directed against the feeble-minded population. One eugenicist contended that '[a]ll available evidence points to the fact that to-day the lower strata of society are far outbreeding the middle and higher, with an almost negligible difference in death-rate, and just in the measure that these lower strata are innately inferior just in that degree must the race deteriorate'.[75] Another added that 'the professional classes are estimated to have had 76% as many children as would suffice for permanent replacement, and the unskilled laborers to have had 117% of the number necessary to replace themselves, after making allowance for differences in mortality'.[76] When such differences were calculated over a number of generations, the results seemed to demonstrate that the moronic lower classes would eventually engulf the entire nation. For many the remarkable fertility of the moron was demonstrated by cases of feeble-minded parents, usually women, with huge numbers of children. Guyer, for example, wrote of a presumably feeble-minded woman who had given birth to twenty-three children,[77] and another writer contended that the average number of children in 'degenerate families' was eleven.[78]

Since the 'degenerate' segment of the population was held to be essentially different from the 'Euro-American' or 'Aryan' type, the race differential argument could not be separated from fears of racial disintegration. This pertained also to the war metaphor since many eugenicists believed that the degenerate population would exact its destruction of society through racial defilement. Britain's Leonard Darwin, the son of Charles, stated flatly that unless eugenic policies were widely implemented, the Western nations would eventually experience the same 'slow and gradual decay' that the previous great cultures had undergone.[79] 'Racial impoverishment', Lothrop Stoddard wrote, 'is the plague of civilization. This insidious disease, with its twin symptoms the extirpation of superior strains and the multiplication of inferiors, has ravaged humanity like a consuming fire, reducing the proudest societies to charred and squalid ruin.'[80] He quoted another eugenicist, who wrote that 'unless we are prepared to cast away the labors of our forefathers and to vanish with the empires of the past, we must accept the office of deciding who are the fittest to prosper and leave offspring'.[81]

Eliminationist rhetoric and eugenics

Few American eugenicists publicly supported euthanasia as a potential measure of eugenic control.[82] Most believed that the primary goal of negative eugenics – that 'defective' persons not breed – would be met just as well by compulsory sterilization as through 'mercy killing'. It was difficult enough for the movement to garner public support for sterilization, let alone for a more controversial measure. In addition, euthanasia and infanticide, if discussed at all, would likely receive widespread support only if they were recommended for the most severely disabled segment of the population, which did not include those labeled as morons.

Nevertheless, the eliminationist rhetoric that was frequently included in eugenic writings was in keeping with the war metaphor as a suitable means of constructing both the public perception of and the nation's response to feeble-mindedness. Lothrop Stoddard said that '[u]nfit individuals as well as unfit social conditions must be eliminated' in order for society to progress,[83] and Karl Schwartz, speaking of the feeble-minded population, asked, 'what general course shall be adopted for their disposal?'[84] Other eugenicists contended that there were 'a good many people living now who ought to have passed away',[85] and discussed the 'elimination of the inherently unfit and anti-social elements of society',[86] the 'necessity of a State eliminating its supply of defectives',[87] and the 'humane elimination' of the unfit.[88] Earnest Hooton said that forced sterilization should at least be allowed for 'specimens of humanity who really ought to be exterminated',[89] and another American eugenicist called for a 'biological house-cleaning' in the nation.[90] Finally, Charles Davenport argued that just as the state or nation had a responsibility to 'deprive the murderer of his life' in order to ensure the protection of innocent persons, 'so also it may annihilate the hideous serpent of hopelessly vicious protoplasm'.[91]

While eugenic writings frequently employed eliminationist rhetoric to undergird calls for restrictive policies and programs, certainly many of those who used such rhetoric would contend that their target was the condition and not the people themselves. In much the same way as we might launch a 'war on cancer' or attempt to 'eradicate AIDS', one could maintain that it is a misinterpretation of these writers to say that their desire was to end the lives of such persons. Taking into account, however, the pejorative view that many had of morons, the degree of social control they supported, and the general feeling of eugenicists that the death of 'unfit' persons was a net benefit to society, there was a very thin line here between the elimination of the condition and the destruction of the persons with the condition.

Feeble-mindedness as a natural catastrophe

Natural catastrophe metaphors were principally used by those in the move-ment to describe the threat of increasing moronity that was occurring as a result of the 'new' immigration from southern and eastern Europe. Obviously one of terms most frequently used to describe the increasing immigrant popu-lation was 'flood', which was potent not only because immigrants traveled over the water, but also because it evoked the image of an inundation and potential submersion that arose from outside the nation's borders.[92] Natural catastrophe metaphors are a likely point of reference in those cases where a particular calamity is considered to be especially descriptive of the impact of the group in question, as is the case here. One immigration restrictionist wrote in 1906 that the 'incoming tide threatens to overwhelm us with the magnitude and ceaseless oncoming of its flood'.[93] If, others warned, limitations were not increased, 'the flood gates will be down and a turgid sea of aliens will inundate our seaports'.[94] James Davis noted that the 1921 restriction law had 'effectively dammed a rising tide of immigration from Europe'.[95] Elizabeth Frazer was particularly picturesque in her description of immigrants:

> It's a ceaseless ebb and flow, a vast tidal river of labor, of homeless peasantry, surging in, surging out, backing up a bit in winters and slack seasons, and boiling out again like a massive sheet of water over a dam at the onset of prosperity in the spring.[96]

Because of the 'flood' of immigrants who were presumed to be feeble-minded or otherwise 'dysgenic', the work of the eugenicists was portrayed by some as a Sisyphean task so long as they focused only on the institutionaliza-tion and sterilization of citizens. Since increasing numbers of immigrants of 'questionable' quality were coming into the country, they argued, these 'inter-nal' methods would have only limited impact. Michael Guyer compared this approach to 'the youth on adventure bent, who was captured by the giant and ... was set the task of sweeping out the giant's stable before sundown'. For just 'as fast as the refuse was swept out at the door an even greater quantity poured in through the windows so that the sweeper, just in proportion to his zeal, became more and more encumbered with his burden'.[97]

Discussion

A central rationale for negative eugenic programs was the contention that uncontrolled moronity was weakening the nation, diverting important resources, exacerbating criminality and other internal disruptive forces, and diluting the blood of the nation. One logical end result of this argument was that the procreation of defectives was making the nation more vulnerable to attack by enemy forces. Eugenicists held that just as Rome and other ancient powers were corrupted from within before they could be successfully occupied, so the United States was weakening itself not only by allowing but more so by actively supporting the propagation of defectives, for example through disease prevention, sanitation, and public assistance measures. Like those who directed their rhetoric at the internal communist conspiracy, many eugenicists believed that the nation would eventually decay from the inside, falling victim to its own inability to limit civil liberties when the good of the country was at stake.

While persons thought to be feeble-minded were presented as a menacing force, however, they were not perceived as conspiratorial or as purposefully attempting to bring down the nation. Indeed, those characteristics that were of greatest concern, their laziness and dependence, hyper-sexuality, criminal behavior, and refusal to live by the values and norms of the community, were all said to arise from an inherent inability as opposed to the conscious decisions that they made. This factor, though, did not diminish the extremity of the threat that they were said to present. Indeed, since they did not understand the harm they posed, eugenicists argued that it was even more important that they be brought under the paternalistic control of the state. Importantly, as is frequently the case, those that were most vociferous in their calls for control of morons and other 'degenerates' were, to a large degree, the same group of professionals who would stand to profit from an expansion in diagnostics, research, institutional development, and the various methods of social control.

At every opportunity, those in the eugenics movement created, nurtured, and disseminated the vision of a once-mighty nation in chaos, with its promise of continued prosperity held hostage by a plight from which only a strong system of negative eugenics could save it. Supporters of this vision would speak ominously of an America that unwittingly empowered its basest and most desperate elements, and subsequently came to be governed by the legion of progeny they would leave in their wake. Eugenicists understood that public sensibilities against the dehumanizing practices that would character-ize eugenic control were much more easily tempered by rationalizations of self-defense than by those of self-betterment. The community which built an institution or acted on its state's sterilization laws was not acting capriciously or with undue malice, but rather was only taking actions that were believed to be necessary to ensure its own survival.

Certainly such rhetoric fell on receptive ears, since the eugenics movement reached its peak as the World War I was being waged. Many were also becoming concerned about the extent to which a specific nation could gain a strategic advantage through a large-scale eugenic program. Eugenicists and military officials also debated the degree to which war might have a 'dysgenic' or 'eugenic' impact on a nation. Many argued for the former position, contending that it was the 'best' males who would become soldiers, and potentially lose their lives. Others, however, said that military conscripts, and especially those who would serve as front-line foot-soldiers, came predominantly from the lower and middle classes, and that their demise would therefore not necessarily have a negative impact on the blood of the nation.

Notes

1 Stoddard, *The Revolt against Civilization*, p. 246.
2 *The International Jew: The World's Foremost Problem*, vol. IV (Dearborn, MI: Dearborn Independent, 1922), pp. 109–10. Also see Zuckier, 'The essential "other" and the Jew'.
3 R.L. Buell, 'The development of anti-Japanese agitation in the United States, II', *Political Science Quarterly* 38 (1923), 65–6.
4 Keen, *Faces of the Enemy*, pp. 76–7.
5 N. Cohn, *Warrant for Genocide: The Myth of the Jewish World-Conspiracy and the Protocols of the Elders of Zion* (New York: Harper & Row, 1966), p. 201. Also see M. Selzer (ed.), *Kike: A Documentary History of Anti-Semitism in America* (New York: World Publishing, 1972).
6 Kevles, *In the Name of Eugenics*, p. 80; Gould, *The Mismeasure of Man*, p. 196.
7 Guyer, *Being Well-Born*, p. 359.
8 Brigham, *A Study of American Intelligence*, pp. 177–81, 182.
9 Barr, 'The imbecile and epileptic *versus* the tax-payer and the community', p. 161; A. Johnson, 'The case of the nation *vs.* the feebleminded', *Survey* 34 (1915), 136–7.
10 A.E. Wiggam, *The Fruit of the Family Tree* (Indianapolis: Bobbs-Merrill Company, 1924), p. 8.
11 Guyer, *Being Well-Born*, p. 405.
12 Stoddard, *The Revolt against Civilization*, pp. 245–6.
13 Johnson, 'The case of the nation', p. 136.
14 Butler, 'The burden of feeble-mindedness', p. 8.
15 J.M. Murdoch, 'Quarantine mental defectives', in *Proceedings of the National Conference on Charities and Correction* (Fort Wayne, IN: Fort Wayne Printing Co., 1909), p. 65.
16 Johnson, 'The case of the nation', p. 137.
17 Such language was also invoked by British eugenicists, including, for example, Charles Darwin's son. See 'Major Darwin predicts civilization's doom unless century brings wide eugenic reforms', *New York Times* (23 August 1932), 16.

18 Quoted in T.W. Shannon, 'Double standard and race degeneracy', *Light* 138 (March–April 1921), 35.

19 Risley, 'Is asexualization ever justifiable in the case of imbecile children?', p. 93.

20 'The future of America: A biological forecast', *Harpers Magazine* 156 (1928), 530.

21 Stoddard, *The Revolt against Civilization*, pp. 240–1.

22 M.W. Barr, 'The prevention of mental defect, the duty of the hour', in *Proceedings of the National Conference on Charities and Correction* (Chicago: Hildmann Printing Co., 1915), p. 361.

23 Quoted in Pernick, *The Black Stork*, p. 95.

24 Barr, 'Mental defectives and the social welfare', p. 747.

25 Goddard, 'The basis for state policy', p. 1852.

26 C.H. Robinson, 'Toward curbing differential births and lowering taxes: A plank or two for eugenic platforms', *Journal of Heredity* 29 (1938), 230.

27 An important element of this fear related to the changing immigration patterns from the 1880s until the 1920s. While immigration into the United States. in the former period was primarily composed of 'Nordics' from northern and western Europe (British, German, French, etc.), by the latter period the vast majority of immigrants were from southern and eastern European nations such as Russia, Romania, and the Baltics. These were, as one might assume, viewed as being less easily assimilated into the country.

28 F.J. Warne, *The Immigrant Invasion*, reprint edn. (New York: American Immigration Library 1971), pp. 2–7.

29 F.F. Weiss, *The Sieve* (Boston: Page Co., 1921), p. 88.

30 Cited in Tucker, *The Science and Politics of Racial Research*, p. 95.

31 Knight, 'Prevention from a legal and moral standpoint', p. 306.

32 Barr, 'The imbecile and epileptic *versus* the tax-payer and the community', p. 163.

33 Kline, *Building a Better Race*, p. 114.

34 Proctor, *Racial Hygiene*, p. 181.

35 Ibid., p. 182.

36 E. Dodge, 'Bettering the birthrates', *Journal of Heredity* 15:3 (1924), 117 (italics in original).

37 Ibid., p. 118.

38 T. Roosevelt, 'Twisted eugenics', *American Motherhood* 38 (1914), 310–11.

39 Guyer, *Being Well-Born*, p. 418.

40 C.B. Davenport, 'The eugenics programme and progress in its achievement', in *Eugenics: Twelve University Lectures* (New York: Dodd, Mead and Company, 1914), p. 12.

41 'Doctor to let patient's baby defective die', p. 2.

42 Quoted in 'U.S. eugenicist hails nazi racial policy', p. 5.

43 Proctor, *Racial Hygiene*, p. 121.

44 Dudziak, 'Oliver Wendell Holmes as a eugenic reformer', p. 861.

45 Ibid. This perception was even more prevalent in Nazi Germany, where medical professionals who helped 'degenerate' persons survive, whereupon they could

eventually propagate, were seen as committing 'treason against the racial heritage of the German people'. See Hitler's *Mein Kampf*, p. 404, and Altman, 'Selection from the skies', p. 134.

46   'Minutes of the Association', p. 23. Also see the similar suggestion quoted by Elks, 'The "lethal chamber"', p. 202.

47   For T.R. Malthus, see his *An Essay on the Principle of Population*, vol. II, reprint edn. (New York: Dutton, 1967).

48   'Eugenics and democracy: A paradox', *Journal of Heredity* 23:5 (1932), 221.

49   Guyer, *Being Well-Born*, p. 356.

50   L. Stoddard, *Racial Realities in Europe* (New York: Charles Scribner's Sons, 1925), p. 102. Also see E.A. Whitney, 'Selective sterilization', *Birth Control Review* 17:4 (1933), 85.

51   S. Humphrey, 'Men and half-men', *Scribners Magazine* 73 (1923), 286–7.

52   '"Biological purge" is urged by Hooton', p. 1.

53   L.F. Whitney, *The Source of Crime*, reprinted from *Christian Work Magazine* by the American Eugenics Society, Inc. (1926).

54   S.J. Holmes, *Human Genetics and its Social Importance* (New York: McGraw-Hill Book Co., Inc., 1936), p. 173.

55   Goddard, *The Kallikak Family*, p. 54.

56   W.E. Fernald, 'The imbecile with criminal instincts', *Journal of Psycho-Asthenics* 14 (1909), 33.

57   'The menace of the feeble-minded', *Eugenical News* 11:2 (1926), 34. For the connection between criminality and feeble-mindedness in Great Britain during the eugenic era, see Jackson's *The Borderland of Imbecility*, p. 108.

58   Kostir, *The Family of Sam Sixty*, p. 28.

59   See, for example, E.H. Johnson, 'Feeble-minded as city dwellers', *Survey* 27 (1912), 1840–3; McKim, *Heredity and Human Progress*, pp. 133, 194; J.T. Mastin, 'The new colony plan for the feeble-minded', in *Proceedings of the National Conference on Charities and Correction* (Chicago: Hildmann Printing Co., 1916), p. 242; 'The menace of the feeble-minded', p. 35.

60   Johnstone, 'Practical provision for the mentally deficient', p. 325.

61   Quoted in M. Lerner (ed.), *The Mind and Faith of Justice Holmes* (Boston: Little, Brown and Company, 1943), p. 358.

62   C. Armstrong, 'The moron menace', *Birth Control Review* 22:5 (1938), 52. For an overview of eugenic writing on the connection between crime and moronity, see L.D. Zeleny, 'Feeble-mindedness and criminal conduct', *American Journal of Sociology* 38 (1933), 564–76. In regard to the framing of mentally ill and mentally retarded persons as criminals in Nazi Germany, see J.M. Gardner, 'Contribution of the German cinema to the Nazi euthanasia program', *Mental Retardation* 20 (1982), 174–5, and E. Slater, 'German eugenics in practice', *Eugenics Review* 27:4 (1936), 289.

63   See, for example, Fernald, 'The feeble-minded', p. 126.

64   For more on 'moral imbecility', see Trent, *Inventing the Feeble Mind*, pp. 84–8.

65 Quoted in S.P. Davies, *Social Control of the Mentally Deficient* (New York: Thomas Y. Crowell Company Publishers, 1930), p. 123.

66 Olson, 'The menace of the half-man', p. 137.

67 Ibid. Also see F. Strother, 'The cause of crime: Defective brain', *World of Work* 48 (1924), 275–86.

68 Fernald, 'The burden of feeble-mindedness', p. 95.

69 See, for example, Guyer, 'Sterilization', p. 36.

70 Malthus, *An Essay on the Principle of Population*, vol. II.

71 W.L. Holt, 'Economic factors in eugenics', *Popular Science Monthly* 83 (1913), 473.

72 Quoted in Stoddard, *The Rising Tide of Color*, p. 256. See also T.J. Curran, *Xenophobia and Immigration, 1820–1930* (Boston: Twayne Publishers, 1975), p. 119; H.H. Laughlin, 'The control of trends in the racial composition of the American people', in M. Grant and C.S. Davison (eds.), *The Alien in Our Midst* (New York: Galton Publishing Co., Inc., 1930), p. 168; K. Young, 'Intelligence tests of certain immigrant groups', *Scientific Monthly* 15 (1922), 418.

73 See, for example, Holt, 'Economic factors in eugenics', p. 474; P. Roberts, *The New Immigration* (New York: Macmillan Company, 1914), p. 346.

74 Laughlin, 'The control of trends', p. 167; See also *Europe as an Immigrant-Exporting Continent*, pp. 1298–9, 1308.

75 Guyer, *Being Well-Born*, p. 419.

76 F. Lorimar, 'Eugenics and birth control', *Birth Control Review* 16:8 (1932), 230. Also see Stoddard, *The Revolt against Civilization*, p. 108.

77 Guyer, 'Sterilization', p. 37.

78 A.W. Wilmarth, 'Report of Committee on Feeble-Minded and Epileptic', in *Proceedings of the National Conference of Charities and Correction* (Boston: Geo. H. Ellis, 1902), p. 154. While the birth differential argument was a prevalent component of eugenic rhetoric in the United States, it was even more apparent within the context of the Nazi program. German race hygienists consistently discussed the 'increasing burden' of the swelling 'degenerate' population, which was especially a concern when considered side by side with the declining birth rate among the non-degenerate 'Aryan' population. See, for example, C. Thomalia, 'The sterilization law in Germany', trans. A. Hellmer, *Eugenical News* 19:6 (1934), 138, and 'Case for sterilization', p. 136.

79 L. Darwin, in 'Echoes of the Eugenics Congress', *Journal of Heredity* 23 (1932), 385–6.

80 Stoddard, *The Revolt against Civilization*, p. 88.

81 Ibid., p. 241.

82 For discussions of euthanasia among American eugenicists, see Hollander's 'Euthanasia and mental retardation: Thinking the unthinkable', *Mental Retardation* 27 (1989), 53–62.

83 Ibid., p. 246.

84 Schwartz, 'Nature's corrective principle in social evolution', p. 85.

85 A.S. Warthin, 'A biologic philosophy or religion a necessary foundation for race betterment', in *Proceedings of the Third Race Betterment Conference* (Battle Creek, MI: Race Betterment Foundation, 1928), p. 86.

86 B. Van Wagenen, 'The eugenic problem', in *Proceedings of the National Conference of Charities and Correction* (Fort Wayne, IN: Fort Wayne Printing Company, 1912), p. 279.

87 Guyer, 'Sterilization', p. 33.

88 Parker, 'The eugenics movement as a public service', p. 345.

89 E.A. Hooton, *Apes, Men and Morons* (New York: G.P. Putnam's Sons, 1937), p. 236.

90 Armstrong, 'The moron menace', p. 53.

91 Davenport, 'Report of Committee on Eugenics', p. 129.

92 See O'Brien, 'Indigestible food, conquering hordes'; W.T. Ellis, 'Americans on guard', *Saturday Evening Post* (25 August 1923), 83; R.D. Ward, 'Eugenic immigration', *American Breeders Magazine* 4:2 (1913), 99.

93 T. Darlington, 'The medico-economic aspect of the immigration problem', *North American Review* 183 (1906), 1266.

94 'Guarding the gates against undesirables', *Current Opinion* 76 (1924), 401.

95 J.J. Davis, 'Jail – or a passport: Some facts and views of immigration', *Saturday Evening Post* (1 December 1923), 134.

96 E. Frazer, 'Our foreign cities: Chicago', *Saturday Evening Post* (25 August 1923), 14.

97 Guyer, *Being Well-Born*, p. 412.

5

THE RELIGIOUS AND ALTRUISTIC METAPHORS: THE MORON AS AN IMMORAL SINNER AND AN OBJECT OF PROTECTION[1]

> Just as none of you would now marry a brother or sister, so you must come to think of it as a crime and a sin – a sin against your race – to marry into a strain that shows feeble-mindedness in its past.[2]

As an integral aspect of modern cultures, religion has often served as an important means of fostering interpersonal bonding, providing hope, direction, and meaning to people and helping to develop a communal sense of morality and demarcate normative from 'deviant' behavior. At times, however, mainstream religious precepts have also served to rationalize the separation of certain subgroups from the community at large, justify social control measures, support existing prejudices, and coerce people to engage in behaviors that run contrary to their own personal self-interest or sense of right and wrong.

Because of religion's central role in society, it is not surprising that religious and spiritual symbols and terminology have frequently been invoked metaphorically. The leaders of social movements attempt to invoke such symbols in order to frame their cause as a religious or spiritual one, or at least present it as compatible with mainstream religious teachings. In many cases religious symbolism or rhetoric will be directly incorporated into propaganda related to the movement and its goals. Efforts may also be made by movement leaders to co-opt religious leaders or networks to communicate issues or proposals, or as a means of highlighting the perceived moral or spiritual foundation of the movement. In nations with a largely Christian population, for example, propagandists will often take pains to demonstrate that Jesus would be supportive of their cause, or that their own leadership is 'Christ-like'. Those who support the cause also may depict themselves as missionaries or prophets, or as sacrificing themselves in some way for the common good. A even Nazi publication referred to the Führer as 'Pope Adolf I', describing him as 'an envoy whom

God has charged with a great mission for his people and for the whole world'.[3] Those who are targeted by various social movements, moreover, are frequently characterized as a demon, anti-Christ, or other specter of evil.

In those societies where freedom of religion is included within the spectrum of individual rights, overt discrimination against those belonging to minority religions is generally deemed to be inappropriate. Even in nations that laud religious freedom, however, persecution may be acceptable, and in some cases may even be presented as a duty. This is especially likely if those who belong to a minority religion, or who profess to be atheists or agnostics, can be perceived as challenging the precepts of the majority religion, and especially if they can be presented as engaging in a conspiracy to damage or destroy it.

Even if target group members are not denigrated on overtly religious grounds, for instance for belonging to a minority religion, religious elements such as immorality or sinfulness often provide a foundation for their depreciation. Groups may be stereotyped as being intemperate, sexually promiscuous, and unfettered by the moral code of the community. In keeping with their sexual immorality, moreover, group members are frequently said to engage in miscegenation and other 'unnatural' sexual behaviors. Writings that supported the segregation of African-Americans, as well as the limitation of Chinese and Japanese immigration, frequently invoked the fear that the male members of these races would mate with white women. Fears of miscegenation and sexual immorality, especially rape, were also predominant in German anti-Semitic propaganda, primarily during the Nazi era, but also prior to the 1930s. For example, one of the principle rationales for refusing to allow Jews to become physicians – or, prior to their removal from the profession, for disallowing them from treating Aryans – was the belief that these physicians were determined to take advantage of non-Jewish female patients.[4]

Many of those who believed in polygenesis or the primordial existence of 'pure races' that had become diluted through intermarriage considered miscegenation to be a hubristic activity that was outside the designs of God. A central tenet of the Great Chain of Being, described in depth in Chapter 3, was that God had created the different species of plants and animals, and that any attempt on the part of humans to control the breeding process by crossing these 'pure' species was a Promethean act doomed to both failure and divine retribution.[5] According to Robert Olby, the taxonomist Carolus Linnaeus had separated 'the species of the Almighty Creator which are true from the abnormal [e.g., hybrid] varieties of the Gardener'. Linnaeus had contended that 'the former persist and have persisted from the beginning of the world', while 'the latter, being monstrosities, can boast but a brief life'.[6] Efforts to disturb the natural order of the system through the breeding of intermediate species, Lovejoy wrote, were often viewed as either 'an act of rebellion against the divine purpose' or a 'crime against Nature'.[7]

When considering the human species specifically, early racial anthropologists such as August De Gobineau and Houston Steward Chamberlain, as well as the earlier supporters of 'manifest destiny' and Anglo-Saxon superiority, placed great stress on the degenerative quality of 'human hybridization'. They pleaded that man should not tinker with the natural workings of nature or God by allowing marriage between those of divergent races or classes.[8] Thus miscegenation fears were buttressed not only by racial arguments, but by religious ones as well.

The altruistic metaphor

An important theme that is prevalent in most efforts to control the rights of marginalized groups has been the argument that such restrictions are in the best interest of those who are to be controlled. Imperialism, for example, was often referred to as the 'white man's burden', implying that those who exerted power and forcibly took over territory and resources were actually sacrificing themselves, as well as providing 'backward' races with protection and the ability to worship the true, Christian God.[9] As noted in Chapter 3, it was said to be the plight of the favored white race to take control over these 'primitive' people and their lands, since such persons were too much like children to take on the responsibility. Encroachments on the part of those in power that are designed to control the behavior of a weaker person or group are often said to be in the best interest of those who are controlled.[10] Albert Wiggam would echo the arguments of earlier racists and social Darwinists in expressing his belief that

> the newer developments in our knowledge of human personality clearly show that some men are contented and happy only when they are oppressed and dominated, provided the dominating is done by the right kind of man. There may be whole races of which this is true, and for whom such a thing as a government operated by the people is not only impossible but the surest way to unhappiness.[11]

Even the most drastic form of social control, large-scale extermination, has been supported by arguing that the action largely results from humanistic regard for the victims. After he assisted in killing a large number of Polish and Russian laborers in the Hadamar asylum,[12] Alfons Klein, an institution administrator, argued in a post-war trial that a majority of these patients were suffering from tuberculosis in its final stage, and arrived here infested with lice and in dirty condition. One must therefore, in judging the facts, differentiate whether healthy, valuable lives were left to die, or whether those who had death stare into their face were given an injection of mercy to relieve them of their incurable and painful suffering.[13]

Supporters of social control measures, then, often argue that they advocate such actions in part because they are in the best interests of the target group members themselves. Often this paternalistic regard for victims easily coexists with concerns that the group is a threatening force that needs to be controlled for the protection of society. Altruistic consideration as a rationale for social control is included in this chapter for several reasons. First, such altruism is often described within a religious context. Control measures may be presented as a form of 'Christian love', charity, or even sacrifice on the part of those who enforce measures of social control. Second, the patronizing attitude that is central to the altruistic metaphor is closely tied to the language of many mainstream religions. The perception of God as a kindly but firm parent figure who lovingly guides and admonishes us is very similar to the way in which authoritarian institutions and groups often present themselves. Lastly, such altruism has frequently been encouraged and employed by religious institutions and leaders.

Eugenic control and the religious metaphor

Many of the authors of secondary works on the subject have referred to the eugenics movement, especially for its most zealous supporters, as a religious endeavor or even a 'secular religion'.[14] Eugenicists themselves often did describe their program as a 'new religion'. Sir Francis Galton, for example, wrote that the subject 'must be introduced into the national conscience, like a new religion'. Eugenics has, he continued, 'strong claims to become an orthodox religious tenet of the future', since it 'co-operate[s] with the workings of nature by securing that humanity shall be represented by the fittest races'.[15] In another work he added that eugenics 'ought to find a welcome home in every tolerant religion', since it 'extends the function of philanthropy to future generations'. Eugenics, he added, was unlike mainstream religions, however, since it 'sternly forbids all forms of sentimental charity that are harmful to the race'.[16]

Interestingly, the first concerted attempt within the United States to improve the species by controlling reproduction took place within a religious community. John Humphrey Noyes's Oneida Community experiment was one of several efforts to develop a 'perfectionist' community during the middle of the nineteenth century.[17] Noyes developed his community in upstate New

York shortly before the American Civil War. Marriage among members was not allowed in the community, and a group of male elders (including Noyes) was given the responsibility of reviewing proposed 'matings' for their potential fitness, as it was assumed that such careful review would give rise to a better class of children. It should come as no surprise that those members who were allowed to have intercourse with the young women of the community were normally the older males who controlled the pairings.[18]

American eugenicists frequently employed religious terminology to describe their goals. Albert Wiggam stated in 1923 that '[e]ugenics means a new religion, new objects of religious endeavor, a new moral code, a new kind of education to our youth, a new conception of many of life's meanings, a new conception of the objectives of social and national life, a new social and political Bible'.[19] Some believed that it could become a 'new religion', surpassing mainstream religions that were not founded on scientific principles of human betterment. Alfred Scott Warthin, for example, the President of the National Association of Physicians, told his audience at the Third Race Betterment Conference that '[o]ld faiths, old superstitions, old beliefs, old emotions' were passing away because of the light of biological research, which was 'a new faith'.[20]

Most eugenicists, however, understood both that their program could be viewed as an act of hubris that infringed on God's domain and that talk of displacing or surpassing Christianity would only diminish its support among the public. They needed to describe their goals rhetorically, then, so that they would be acceptable to the public and seem congruent with existing religious precepts. Most, then, contended that they were acting in conjunction with God's plans. When speaking of eugenics as a 'new religion', they clearly meant that their goal was not to surpass or replace Christianity, but rather to improve man's spiritual standing by improving man. In assisting the evolution of humans in a 'desirable' direction, eugenicists argued that they were creating a more perfect race, which certainly must be in line with divine intent and conventional religious teachings. 'God', Leon Whitney wrote in 1926, 'loves perfection. This great strain which God or nature developed by the kindly selective process was no doubt much greater than the race from which it sprang and must have been very dear unto God.'[21] In helping to foster this more perfect species, eugenicists argued, they were 'apostles of a social ethics'.[22]

Many eugenicists who held a social Darwinist perspective contended that if 'encroaching on God's realm' was a primary reason for opposing eugenic policies, the development of medical, public health, and other environmental and social reform measures that kept alive persons who previously would have perished could also be viewed as subverting divine intent. In counteracting

these unnatural preservation measures, not by killing the unfit, but simply by
ensuring that they would not breed, eugenicists argued, they were serving to
keep the stock from becoming not only physically but also morally 'polluted'.
As Walter Hadden wrote in 1914:

> The world can not go on deteriorating, and degenerating without ruining the
> designs of God that man shall aim for the highest things in life. Nowhere can
> it be found that the Almighty while insisting upon reproduction, insists that it
> shall be carried on without reason and common sense ... To reach perfection
> was the constant insistence of Christ. In the Sermon on the Mount, addressing
> the multitude he said: 'Be ye therefore perfect, even as your Father which is in
> heaven is perfect'. There is no justification here for perpetuating imperfection,
> but the contrary.[23]

Jesus as eugenicist

As Hadden's statement demonstrates, a number of those who wrote in support
of the movement assured their readers that Jesus himself would back their
measures. Albert Wiggam declared that '[h]ad Jesus been among us, he would
have been president of the First Eugenics Congress',[24] and that '[s]cience
came not to destroy the great ethical essence of the Bible but to fulfill it'.[25]
Other supporters of eugenic control noted that Jesus 'was born into the world
without any hereditary taint', that this physical and mental normalcy 'is what
he craved for every other child of God',[26] and that it 'lies within the purpose
of God that every life born into the world should grow up tall and straight and
should be clean and pure'.[27] Moreover, just as Jesus had sacrificed himself for
the good of the world, eugenicists invested the concept into their own writings, contending that unfit persons needed to sacrifice themselves, by resisting
their carnal urges, for the overall good of society.[28]

Biblical verses, especially the teachings of Jesus, were frequently invoked
as examples to demonstrate that eugenic measures were in keeping with the
principles of Christianity. Leon Whitney, for example, described the parable
of the sower as analogous to eugenics. A man who sowed good seeds in his
field came to find that weeds also had grown up, the latter being the product
of an enemy who 'came and sowed tares among the wheat' while the owner
slept. When harvest came, the wheat was to be gathered and placed into barns,
while the 'bad seed' was to be burned to ensure that it would no longer grow.
Whitney concluded that in following out this injunction, church leaders must
join forces with eugenicists and 'do their part in seeing that the seed from the
human tares does not go over into the next generation'.[29] To Wiggam, eugenics was little more than an updated version of the Golden Rule. The 'biological

Golden Rule', he said, was to '[d]o unto both the born and the unborn as you would have both the born and the unborn do unto you'.[30] The book that contained this quotation, The New Decalogue of Science, referred to an updated, more scientifically focused version of the Ten Commandments, with, Christine Rosen wrote, the New Mount Sinai being the laboratory.[31]

According to Christine Rosen, who explored the relationship between eugenic writing and religion in her book Preaching Eugenics, the medals given to winners of 'Fitter Families' contests included an inscription from Psalm 16: 'Yea, I have a goodly heritage'.[32] Rosen contended that the American Eugenics Society purposefully included Christian symbolism in its eugenics propaganda in part to recruit religious leaders to support its cause.[33] Irving Fisher, a Yale professor, said of birth control as a eugenic measure that, like the Biblical flood, it could be a 'means first of wiping out the old world and then replacing it by a new'.[34] Earnest Hooton too borrowed the Biblical flood metaphor, arguing that humankind was like Noah and the ark, and that 'the deluge is upon us'.[35] Implicit in this reference was that those chosen to be in the ark needed to be not the most moral or religious, but the most 'eugenically fit'. Of course, to the majority of eugenicists, these were one and the same.

A partnership with the churches

Davenport, Laughlin, and leaders of the movement called on mainstream churches and ministers not only to support but also to take a prominent role in the movement. In 1926 the Eugenical News announced that the American Eugenics Society was holding a competition for those preachers who could best incorporate the issue of eugenics into their sermons. This competition was open to ministers and theological students from all demominations, and the society also printed a 'Eugenics Catechism' and formed a 'Committee on Cooperation with Clergymen'.[36] Both the eugenic sermon competition and the committee met with success, although, according to Rosen, religious leaders responded to the 'social message of eugenics rather than its scientific details'.[37] Their goal was not to subvert the mainstream religious institutions, eugenicists said, but rather to work with the churches to lead their flocks to become closer to God. Many in the United States movement would certainly have agreed with the British eugenicists Whetham and Whetham, who wrote:

> Of late years the Christian Church has organized much of its social work on a revised sense of the old conception of the brotherhood of man. We must now look to it to lead a movement in another direction, even more deeply fraught with spiritual meaning, where parenthood and responsibility to those who will follow after us will be the uniting principles of new religious life.[38]

Ministers, priests, and other clerics and religious leaders were especially desirable allies for those in the eugenics movement because of their roles in facilitating marriage bonds. Since an important goal of the movement was to ensure that prospective mates had considered each other's hereditary fitness prior to marriage, and many eugenicists fought for state laws that would restrict marriage among the 'unfit', they also realized that the cooperation of those who administered marriages was essential. Even without such legislation, some members of the clergy, led by Walter Sumner, decided to refuse to marry couples unless they could produce health certificates providing evidence that they did not have a hereditary or communicable disease.[39]

According to Rosen, a large number of clerics, especially liberals with a social reform outlook, took up Sumner's call to marry only couples who could demonstrate 'fitness'. The Progressivist focus on prevention and amelioration of disease and social problems had an important influence in many Protestant churches, and a large number of religious leaders, like Sumner, believed they could help usher in 'the Kingdom of God on earth through reform and service'.[40] Many eugenicists, while applauding these ministers for recognizing the importance of eugenic control, were lukewarm in their support of the certificates, primarily because they believed that they would be of limited benefit, since they were certain that morons would likely procreate whether married or not.[41]

Some eugenicists additionally called the Catholic Church to task for its celibacy policy. They held that those who fell under the policy were presumably physically fit, well-educated, and pious individuals. To deny such prospective parents the opportunity to have children was seen as highly dysgenic. According to Huntington and Whitney:

> We wonder that the Holy Father of the Roman Catholic Church does not go up into the mountain and view his world in the light of eugenics. We should think a farmer either crazy or hopelessly stupid if he continually killed off his best animals and let the poorer do the breeding. Yet that is what religious celibacy, as now practiced, does to the human race.[42]

Religious metaphors and euthanasia

The small number of American eugenicists who supported euthanasia as a viable control measure attempted to find religious rationales to buttress their positions. In discussing Dr Haiselden's refusal to treat the Bollinger baby in 1915, a physician wrote, '[t]he human body, we are told, is the temple of the living God'. A body like that 'of the babe in question', he continued, 'would be a poor receptacle for the indwelling Holy Spirit'.[43] A minister who supported

Haiselden's decision wrote that medical interventions to extend the life of such children were 'forbidding the children to go to [God] when He calls'.[44] Foster Kennedy, a physician and a principal supporter of passive euthanasia, likewise said in 1939 that a primary concern of legalizing the measure was that even the severely disabled or comatose had 'immortal souls'. Kennedy contended that even if this was true, 'to release that soul from its misshapen body which only defeats in this world the soul's powers and gifts is surely to exchange, on that soul's behalf, bondage for freedom'.[45] Karl Schwartz contended that aiding 'nature in her task of elimination' was in conjunction with 'the best interpretation of Christian ethics'.[46] 'It was not God', Huntington and Whitney wrote in 1927, 'who made the defectives. *We* made them, or our forefathers did. God kills them off, for that is Nature's stern way; we make them by disregarding the laws of heredity, by preserving the weak and imbecile, and by making it easy for defectives to reproduce their kind.'[47] This relationship between euthanasia and religious rhetoric will be taken up again below in the section on altruism.

Sin, virtue, and human reproduction

Religious rhetoric was frequently used to describe the breeding of both 'fit' and 'unfit' persons. While 'eugenic' matings were described as virtuous, dysgenic couplings, which presumably fostered the hereditary transmission of degenerative characteristics, were said to be grievous sins against society. Martin Barr discussed eugenic marriages as a great and noble virtue:

> [the] sacred entrance to the vocation of parenthood to which all are not called; a vocation for which the fitting of oneself by the cultivation of the being – mental, moral and physical – toward the gaining of a noble self-hood is the truest religion as well as following the dictates of the highest patriotism. Such preservation of things sacred would lead, surely, to a day of chivalry greater than that of past ages.[48]

In opposition to 'sacred' eugenic marriages, however, dysgenic marriage (or reproduction) was profane. Even before the turn of the century, Kate Wells had written that '[t]he marriage of deaf-mutes is [a] "physiological sin", as such crimes have been well termed'.[49] The Canadian physician and advocate of eugenics Helen MacMurchy added that it was a 'sacrilege' that the 'holy duties' of motherhood, which was the highest of all professions, were profaned by allowing feeble-minded women to have children.[50] She added, several pages later, that it was a 'sin' to allow feeble-minded persons 'to raise up children in their likeness, as we now do'.[51] Aldred Warthin, a pathologist and early

cancer researcher, contended that 'theological terms' provided an apt means
of describing eugenics. In discussing 'biological sins', he wrote that 'our biologic mission is to carry on this immortal stream of germ plasm', and that any
healthy person who refused to bring children into the world was committing a
grave biological sin.[52] As will be further described below, it was in their role as
sexual transgressors that morons were especially held up as 'sinners'.

Eugenicists frequently referred to 'unfit' persons, and especially the feeble-
minded, as evil entities or a principal source of evil in the world. In her book
Race Improvement or Eugenics, LaReine Baker called racial degeneration 'the
scientists' formula for the theologian's "fall from grace"',[53] and wrote that the
'eugenist does not say that religion, morality, and education are ineffective, he
only claims that these great forces should apply to the foundations of society
instead of being spent and dissipated in a thousand less important directions'.[54]
Some even described feeble-minded persons as 'incubuses' or demon spirits.
In the home such children were said to be 'an incubus upon the unhappy
mother'.[55] Misguided philanthropy, another writer intoned, served to 'burden
the future with an incubus of mental deficiency'.[56] Lydia DeVilbiss argued that the
belief that many had previously held that feeble-minded and other 'defective'
children were the result of divine retribution upon sinful parents was a myth.
Nevertheless, she added, such children were indeed the natural result of 'igno-
rance or sin'. It was not God, however, who was responsible for the result, but
rather the parents, who had not employed eugenic standards when choosing a
mate and deciding to have children.[57]

In 1934 Dr Theodore Robie, a strong supporter of eugenic control, discussed the case of the daughter of a mentally defective father who 'contracted
gonorrhea at eight and a half years as a result of a supposed rape by a man of
fifty-two'. Did Dr Robie express outrage at this rape of a child of eight and a
half? Quite the contrary: he assumed that 'considering her low mental capacity it is more than probable that she made little effort to prevent this assault'.[58]
While being an extreme example, this statement is indicative of the effort that
was made throughout the eugenic period to portray the moron as the primary
source of sexual immorality within the nation. In the context of eugenic
propaganda, males were likely to take advantage of young children or feeble-
minded women, and the females were sure to become prostitutes and to bear
large numbers of illegitimate progeny. Members of both genders were almost
certain to engage in sexual activity outside marriage, often with multiple part-
ners, and feeble-minded persons were also apt to become sexually active with
those of a different race. In their presumed hyper-sexuality morons stood out
as not only consummate sinners, but moreover as persons who were apt to
lead others into evil.[59]

It was especially the female moron who was considered to be sexually perverted and, as noted in Chapter 2, a principal source of societal pollution. Many eugenicists were obsessed with the reputed sexual exploits of the female moron. They took for granted that such women were easily led astray by males in search of easy sexuality without commitment. Gosney and Popenoe, strong advocates of female sterilization, wrote that the woman who was committed to an institution as feeble-minded was 'characteristically a sex delinquent'. Such a woman, they said, was 'oversexed, feebly inhibited, lacks other interests, and is not merely a ready prey to unscrupulous males, but too often herself an aggressor in this field'.[60] If a feeble-minded woman became involved with males whose intellectual ability was unknown or 'normal', it was often assumed that the woman was at fault, as the males 'otherwise would not have been led into vicious habits'.[61]

As Dugdale noted about the Juke women, prostitution in female morons was taken to be the gender equivalent of criminality in the males.[62] Eugenic writings were teeming with statistics of the reputedly high number of prostitutes who were classified as feeble-minded. The sweeping immorality of such people was also supported by cases of 'moron' women who had borne extraordinarily high numbers of children.[63] The supposed sexual immorality of the female moron, moreover, was exploited to provide a ready explanation for genealogical research results that did not fit eugenic presuppositions. A core belief of many early eugenicists, for example, was that two feeble-minded parents could not have a 'normal' child. When such an occurrence came to pass, writers simply assumed that the mother, unable to control her sexual behavior, had engaged in an extramarital affair with a non-feeble-minded man, who was thus the genetic father of the child.[64] According to Goddard,

> When we consider the social status and moral habits of most of the families in which hereditary feeble-mindedness occurs, we must recognize that there will always be some uncertainty as to parentage. A feeble-minded woman married to a feeble-minded man and giving birth to a normal child, may possibly be an instance where the husband of the wife is not the father of the child.[65]

Like a contemporary Eve or Pandora,[66] the wayward female was seen as the source of degeneracy in most eugenic family studies. The Kallikaks had their feeble-minded bar-maid whose dalliance with Martin Kallikak senior supposedly began the dysgenic line,[67] and the Jukes were traced to the six Juke sisters, including 'Margaret, the mother of criminals'.[68] Gertrude Davenport said that a man's 'marriage with a woman of wandering and vicious disposition' was the reason for the 'permanent downfall' of the degenerate branch of a European family that she described.[69] Writers of family studies were especially likely to note when miscegenation had taken place within these families, as it was often contended that this 'racial sin' began or exacerbated the families' decline.[70] For example, Michael Guyer noted that the 'Tribe of Ishmael', a 'degenerate' Indiana family, was the result of 'the progeny of a neurotic man and a half-breed woman'.[71]

As with both Deborah Kallikak and Carrie Buck, it was largely the fear of sexual promiscuity, or the birth of a child out of wedlock, that would precipitate efforts to forcibly segregate or sterilize females classed as morons or 'high-grade' imbeciles. If such a woman, Popenoe and Johnson wrote, 'had behaved herself she would have been kept at home in many instances'.[72] As Kline noted, normality – and therefore also moronity – was defined as much by 'moral purity' as it was by 'mental capacity'.[73] In fact, she wrote, as the sterilization movement evolved, sexual immorality came to be considered, at least in some states, a more important rationale for the procedure than the diagnosis of a hereditary impairment.[74]

Besides intercourse that would lead to pregnancy or venereal disease, other forms of 'immoral' sexuality were derided by eugenicists. Especially early in the movement, masturbation was a target of control and a primary rationale for the castration of institutionalized residents, even after the development of the vasectomy. 'Self-abuse', Risley wrote in 1905, aggravated 'the nervous disorders already existing' among the feeble-minded. It was also 'held to be an important etiologic factor in epilepsy and deranged mental states'. Therefore, he concluded, to 'remove from the imbecile this vicious tendency would in many cases render him or her more docile and amendable to efficient training. Their general health would improve and their lives, in some measure, be lifted from the slough of degradation.'[75] In his book *The Unfit*, Elof Carlson described the efforts during the nineteenth century, in the United States as well as Europe, to deal effectively with the 'disease' of masturbation.[76] As one might expect, the condition was especially considered to be prevalent among groups whose alternative sexual outlets were diminished and who were under frequent surveillance by others. This would include, of course, the residents of institutions for the feeble-minded.

Many observers felt that a high rate of alcoholism also exacerbated the sexual problems of morons. Just as studies were said to demonstrate that a large percentage of prostitutes, paupers, and criminals were feeble-minded, they did the same with drunkards. Walter Fernald discussed a British study which found that 'seventy per cent of the habitual drunkards who are dealt with under the Inebriate Act are mentally defective'.[77] However, as Marouf Hasian wrote, some eugenicists actually opposed prohibition, arguing that this would run counter to social Darwinism, since 'alcohol was a selective agent for killing off the unfit'.[78]

As noted in the previous chapter, eugenic goals were, in general, commensurate with the objectives of the social purity movement of the late nineteenth and early twentieth centuries. This campaign appealed to both Progressivists and moral conservatives, and counted among its goals the decrease and eventually elimination of smoking, drinking, illicit sex, venereal disease, and prostitution, along with a promulgation of community and individual health and sanitation measures. While many of these goals are euthenic, requiring community reform, eugenicists argued that only a combination of euthenic and eugenic approaches would curb the immorality that was sweeping the nation, especially since so many of these social problems were attributed to inherited moronity.

The altruistic metaphor and eugenic control

The contention that persons with feeble-mindedness benefitted from and, in many cases, even desired measures of control (or would have if they could make a 'reasoned' decision) was a principal theme of eugenic writings. Institutionalization, sterilization, and other restrictive policies, these writings held, not only would protect society from the burdensome weight of future morons, but also were in keeping with the public's Christian duty to provide for and protect such unfortunates who could not live on their own and were constantly threatened by the dangers of their environment. Thus discussions regarding the proper course of care given to feeble-minded persons were filled with paternalistic arguments that presented institutional administrators and other authorities as benevolent care-givers who were sacrificing their time to protect morons and provide them with a higher quality of life than they otherwise could be expected to have. To quote J. David Smith:

> Eugenics programs have often been proposed in ways that make them appear to be not only for the good of society but also for the good of the victim. I suspect that in some cases the proposers of such measures sincerely believed that they were looking out for the best interests of the inferior. In any case, from the Kallikaks onward, eugenic actions have often been presented as being 'for their own good': The retarded should be institutionalized for their own protection. They should be sterilized so that they can be released. They should be allowed a 'good death' so that they do not have to bear the pain of a 'life devoid of meaning'.[79]

Lothrop Stoddard agreed that while social control policies were 'stern toward bad *stocks*', toward the individuals who comprised these 'stocks' they were characterized by their kindness and 'profound humaneness'.[80] It was not unusual for those who carried out eugenic policies to characterize their work as similar to 'missionary work',[81] and they described themselves as 'devoted and self-sacrificing men and women'.[82] Before the turn of the century, John Broomall, an eminent judge from Pennsylvania, wrote that there were some groups who thrived when placed under the strict supervision of responsible persons:

> The Indian, the lunatic, the imbecile, the public enemy, submits to the law of kindness. The wayward child obeys those who love it. Even wild beasts are subject to this law. The successful lion-tamer is the man who loves the lion, and his first lesson is to teach the pupil that he loves it.[83]

Eugenicists considered feeble-minded persons to have the mentality of children,[84] and that their rights could thus be controlled in the same way as a child's rights are. What Wolf Wolfensberger termed the 'perpetual child' metaphor[85] has frequently been employed over the years to not only characterize persons with mental disabilities but moreover to rationalize the restriction of their rights, and at no time was this more apparent than during the eugenic alarm era. This is especially problematic since it was not idiots and imbeciles who were targeted for involuntary segregation and sterilization, but rather the 'higher-functioning' moron class. Martin Barr justified segregation by stating that 'we are dealing not with men, but with an arrested development which constitutes a perpetual childhood'.[86] A principal role of the state, then, was to help keep such persons 'innocent, as little children are innocent'.[87] According to Leila Zenderland, Henry Goddard, like other eugenicists, viewed persons with cognitive disabilities as previous supporters of manifest destiny perceived the 'primitive' peoples of non-Western cultures: as intellectual and emotionally immature beings who required guidance from responsible others.[88] She adds that Goddard, who provided expert testimony in a few death penalty cases, was disturbed by fact that some feeble-minded persons in the community who had committed crimes were sentenced to death. He believed that since these persons had the mentality of children, they should be institutionalized rather than killed.[89]

Many eugenicists, especially institutional administrators, argued that it was only within a properly run institution that morons would be able to enjoy happy and care-free lives.[90] Such facilities, Barr wrote, served a dual purpose, benefitting both society and the individual: '[s]ociety must be protected from pollution and tragedy on the one hand, and on the other the innocent imbecile must be saved from punishment for heedless or reckless transgression for which he is absolutely irresponsible'.[91] Over a decade later he asked why a reservation was not set aside for the feeble-minded, since they were 'as deserving' of one as were 'the Indian or the Negro'.[92] While forced institutionalization, he noted in the same article, had earlier been viewed as a form of brutality, it was now looked upon as 'the safeguarding of the innocent'.[93] Sanborn, writing in support of the state's use of its commitment powers under the *parens patriae* (state as parent) doctrine, suggested that '[t]he strong arm of the state should extend its protection to the absolutely helpless as well as to those suffering from slight mental enfeeblement'.[94] Alexander Johnson invoked the teachings of Jesus in calling for the segregation of feeble-minded children as a means of protecting them:

> the Master said that it was better for us to have a mill-stone around our necks and to be cast into the depths of the sea, than that we should cause one of these little ones to offend, or that we should offend one of these little ones. And when we as a people either by laws or by absence of laws, expose these little ones to wrong and shame, we are incurring that condemnation ... The attitude of the state should be that of a good and loving mother to them.[95]

Among other benefits of segregation, it would presumably allow feeble-minded persons to associate with their 'own kind', who would not make fun of them or exploit their weaknesses, and it would protect them from the temptations of the outside world, to which they, because of their lack of control, could not resist succumbing. Furthermore, since they could assist with the labor of the institution, they would be useful and engage in wholesome and supervised occupation. By helping with the 'lower-grade' students, the morons could even fill a minor care-giver role, which would especially be beneficial to the females, but also to the males.[96] It was perhaps, the 'most touching' sight in the facility, Alexander Johnson said, 'to see the tenderness and patience exercised by a great, big, overgrown man-baby toward a tiny child-baby, when put into his care. Here is a place which the imbecile can fill, often as well as and certainly more willingly than a hired helper.'[97] Moreover, by working in the institution, morons would not be 'subject to the strain of free competition within the community'.[98]

Since many eugenicists felt that feeble-mindedness was primarily heredi-tary, they assumed that many feeble-minded children lived with parents of a similar mentality who could not take care of them, or were abusive or neglectful. The institution, then, would protect these children from those within their own family circle who wanted to mistreat or take advantage of them.[99] For those parents who were neither abusive nor themselves feeble-minded, removal of the child from the home would, eugenicists promised, reduce the burden on the family and would allow the parents to focus atten-tion on their other children, who could actually make a future for themselves. Institutionalization, therefore, was beneficial not only to the resident, but to the family as well.

Eugenicists contrasted the quality of life of those who were residing in institutions with that of their 'peers' who were out in the community. Discussing the relatives of Deborah Kallikak who were still living in rural New Jersey, Leila Zenderland noted that '[i]n their ragged clothing and shabby surroundings' they were presented in Goddard's writings as 'a pitiful sight'. Their poor state, moreover, was especially apparent when their lot was compared with that of the more fortunate Deborah, who was '[p]hotographed in a lovely dress, a big bow in her hair, a book in her hands, and a cat lying contentedly across her lap'.[100] She had, in other words, been saved from a life of squalor by the beneficence of institutional officials. Only within a segregated setting, advocates wrote, would feeble-minded persons truly have 'a happy, smiling existence'.[101] Johnstone wrote of the moron that 'in his village of the simple, this land of eternal childhood, he finds joy and gladness'.[102]

Just as sexual segregation was rationalized as being in the best interest of the morons as well as the society at large, so was sterilization. It is certainly ironic, then, that one of the principal benefits that eugenicists touted for sterilization was that it would allow persons to leave the institution. Even before the development of the vasectomy and salpingectomy, Martin Barr supported the castration of some of his charges, since it would allow them to live in the community.[103] Other advocates of eugenics described their support of these more invasive procedures as beneficial to those who were subject to them. Prior to the development of the tubal ligation, for example, Isaac Kerlin allowed one of the residents in the Pennsylvania Training School to have her 'procreative organs' removed. This, he contended, 'has been her salvation from vice and degradation'. In a nod to the philanthropic beneficiary who paid for the operation, Kerlin added that he was 'deeply thankful to the benevolent lady whose loyalty to science and comprehensive charity made this operation possible'.[104]

In Great Britain in 1910, Winston Churchill, then the British Home Secretary, supported calls for a national eugenic sterilization policy, contending that it 'was a merciful act' since it was 'cruel to shut up numbers of people in institutions for their whole lives, if by a simple operation they could be permitted to live freely in the world without causing much inconvenience to others'.[105] In the *Buck* case, the Virginia Appeals Court noted that the procedure was not a punishment, but rather was designed to 'protect the class of socially inadequate citizens named therein from themselves'.[106]

The procedure itself was described by eugenicists as 'humane', 'minor', 'trivial', and a 'simple and harmless' practice.[107] Most operations were 'not performed under duress and legal pressure', Albert Wiggam wrote, 'but are merely instituted through persuasion of the individuals on the part of tactful physicians and prison officials'.[108] He added that it was neither a punishment nor a cruel method of control. It was, he said, 'not nearly so severe a surgical interference as removing tonsils or pulling abscessed teeth'.[109]

Supporters argued that sterilization not only helped morons by ensuring that they would not be saddled with children whom they could not properly raise, but in many cases actually helped change poor attitudes or behaviors. Whitney and Shick said that many of those who underwent the procedure would "'brighten up" considerably mentally and the majority seem more easily managed and less temperamental'.[110] These authors displayed several graphs showing the improvement in habits exhibited by residents following operations.[111] Eugenicists lauded the 'therapeutic value' of sterilization,[112] and noted that the procedure was the 'kindest' way of 'aiding the feeble-minded'.[113] A Kansas physician who performed sterilizations for the state contended that many additional persons should have 'the benefit of this operation'.[114] According to Paul Weindling, a sex counselor in Frankfurt said, shortly before the Nazis gained power, that she believed sterilization 'had a rejuvenating effect' on many people.[115]

Advocates of sterilization frequently noted that those who were subject to the operations were among its biggest supporters. Eugenicists argued that 'the sterilized patients themselves are often greatly pleased, with the results',[116] that 'even those who have been sterilized are … enthusiastically friendly to the measure',[117] and that most of those 'sterilized either welcome the operation or make no objection to having it performed'.[118] Those in institutions who might be released if sterilized, LeBourdais wrote, saw sterilization as 'a badge of distinction'.[119] Paul Popenoe and E.S. Gosney, two leaders of California's race betterment program, were especially outspoken in arguing that sterilized patients were not only helped by the measure, but highly supportive of it. Of the hundreds of patients they spoke to after being sterilized, only a handful, they said, were displeased. They noted that for many, especially the women, the procedure, even when involuntarily applied, gave them a sense of relief that 'outweighs the feeling of loss of children'.[120] Many of the women they interviewed were 'pathetic in their expression of gratitude' and expressed their desire that others in such circumstances would 'have the same protection'.[121] For the small number of disgruntled patients, especially those diagnosed as either feeble-minded or insane, the authors placed the blame not on the coercive nature of the procedure, but rather on the person's 'abnormal' condition; 'since many of these persons are still more or less disturbed mentally', they said, 'it might have been expected that they would find this as good an excuse as any to give vent to the feelings of persecution which animate many of the victims of such diseases'.[122]

Some admitted, however, that a primary reason for the support of patients was the promise of freedom that it offered them. For example, Mary Dudziak wrote that Dr Priddy, a physician involved in the *Buck v. Bell* case, had said that 'feeble-minded women "clamor for" eugenical sterilization "Because they know what it means for enjoyment of life and the peaceful pursuance of happiness, as they view it, on the outside of institution walls"'.[123]

The small number of American eugenicists who openly supported euthanasia too often used sugar-coated language to describe 'mercy killing'. William Lennox, a Harvard neurologist, spoke of the 'privilege of death for the congenitally mindless',[124] and another physician, William Duncan McKim, said that:

> The surest, the simplest, the kindest, and most humane means for preventing reproduction among those whom we deem unworthy of this high privilege, is a *gentle, painless death*; and this should be administered not as a punishment, but as an expression of enlightened pity for the victims – too defective by nature to find true happiness in life – and as a duty toward the community and toward our own offspring.[125]

Huntington and Whitney discussed the case of a child of a prostitute who was born 'badly afflicted with a loathsome venereal disease'.[126] While social workers had taken the child to the hospital, they wondered whether it would be more 'merciful and charitable' to help the child to die. Then, they said, the 'poor, miserable, sickly little thing ... would have been saved from years of torture'.[127] Similarly, in *The Black Stork*, an early film supporting Harry Haiselden's infanticide cases, the mother of a 'severely disabled' baby requires surgery to save its life. The physician, who is actually played by Haiselden, refuses to operate. The mother 'is torn by uncertainty until God reveals a lengthy vision of the child's future, filled with pain, madness, and crime'. Thus she relents and allows the child to die, and in the next scene 'the baby's soul leaps into the arms of a waiting Jesus'.[128] Martin Pernick wrote that 'Haiselden compared the Bollinger baby to the Christ child, explaining that the infant's sacrifice revealed a new rationally based testament to supercede the old religion'.[129]

Numerous writers have discussed the lengths to which German eugenicists went to argue that their own euthanasia program was in the best interests of its victims.[130] Such rhetoric predated the Nazis. For example, in their 1920 book supporting euthanasia for persons with mental disabilities, Binding and Hoche referred to it as 'act of healing'[131] and a way of 'rescuing so many incurables from their suffering'.[132] The language of 'release', 'salvation', 'special treatment', and 'deliverance' was frequently employed by the Nazis in discussing the program, and such terms often served as 'code words' within official memoranda. A condolence letter sent to the family of a victim of the program noted that his death – from a fabricated cause[133] – 'delivered him from his suffering and spared him from institutionalization for life'.[134] Advocates noted that those who did not support euthanasia were forcing thousands of 'hopeless' individuals to endure unimaginable suffering,[135] and the films commissioned by the Reich to lend support to the programs focused heavily on the great kindness of ending such suffering[136] and the benefit of 'removing a burden' from afflicted families.[137]

Supporters of eugenics in the United States and elsewhere argued that not only were their proposed measures beneficial to those who were targeted by them, but they also helped those not yet born. Since it was a 'serious matter to bestow life' on an individual with a heritable disease, or to force upon them unfit parents, preventing such lives from coming into being was described as an important side benefit of eugenic programs.[138] Eugenicists frequently talked of the child's right to good parents or the 'right to be well-born',[139] and Goddard contended that it would be better for morons had they 'never been born'.[140] Supporters contended that one of the principal duties of the eugenics movement was to press for policies that would ensure that future children did not suffer by being born with a disabling condition. 'I plead on behalf of the unborn', a British eugenicist wrote, 'of the infants and children of the future – "the coming race" – and against our present Christian custom of stamping the unoffending child with a mental defect that will prevent it from being a useful citizen'.[141] Jessie Taft, a leading scholar in the burgeoning social work profession, added that controlling the propagation of the unfit was an important means of protecting 'future generations' from injury,[142] and Leon Cole added that 'the desire to prevent suffering must extend to the desire to prevent the suffering of unborn generations'.[143]

As one might guess, few of those who justified eugenic measures as a means of protecting future persons from suffering took note of the fact that these persons would not exist at all if such policies were passed. For those 'future children' on whose behalf the eugenicists acted as advocates, the issue was not a choice between living without a 'hereditary illness' and living with one, but rather whether it was better to live with such a condition or to not live at all.

Discussion

Any person, group, or institution that advocates for the systematic control of human breeding must deal with prevailing social fears that the methods they support supersede organized religious precepts and therefore constitute acts of hubris. This is true not only of eugenics as it was practiced in the first half of the century, but of contemporary genetic advancements as well. As Charles Frankel wrote decades before the human genome was mapped,

> There hovers about biomedicine the scent of ancient taboos broken, of entry into forbidden territory. It stirs to life fears that go back to the oldest myths in our civilization, and revives religious attitudes about sin, trespass, and tinkering with the delicate harmonies of the Creation that lie just below the level of consciousness even in agnostics and atheists.[144]

Since eugenics deals with the elemental structure and composition of individuals and groups and seeks to change this composition in profound ways, it has often been viewed as an intrusion on the designs of God.

The employment of religious rhetoric within the context of the eugenic alarm period had the primary purpose of demonstrating that controlled human breeding was in keeping with the teachings of Christianity. The logic of eugenicists was clear. If God was perfect, and wanted humans to become as much like him as possible, the perfectibility of man was not only permissible but a divine mandate. This was especially true, they argued, since through medical and public health advancements and other means of social reform, humans had effectively overturned the natural or divinely ordained agents of evolution. Similarly, the eugenicists picked up on the Great Chain of Being's tenet that those humans who were the most perfect had the greatest affinity to God. Therefore, physical, spiritual, and mental improvement were portrayed as the most reliable ways of coming into the good graces of the Lord. Additionally, how could one reconcile, eugenicists wondered, the knowledge that man was created in God's image with the existence of persons who were severely disfigured or disabled? Efforts to reconcile the presence of feeble-minded, insane, and other disabled individuals with the designs of God and mainstream religious teachings have been long-standing.[145]

It was during the eugenic era that persons who were thought to have intellectual impairments were first widely viewed as sexual beings. While idiots and 'lower-functioning' imbeciles continued to be considered 'eternal children' or 'holy innocents', to use Wolf Wolfensberger's phrases,[146] morons and 'higher-functioning' imbeciles such as Carrie Buck (especially the females) were presented as the sexual antithesis of the idiot. They were portrayed as hypersexual beings whose immoral behavior threatened the moral underpinnings of the community, and as a source of not only physical but indeed spiritual pollution.

While it was obviously Hitler's eugenics that most clearly integrated Nietzsche's philosophy into the sphere of controlled breeding, an undercurrent of Nietzscheism can certainly be seen in the arguments of American eugenicists. When the German philosopher wrote in *Thus Spoke Zarathustra* that God had died, he added that the reason for God's death was his pity for man.[147] In other words, by refusing to allow the poor, weak, and disfigured to die out, God (and, by association, mainstream Christianity) had become 'soft' and thus ensured that humans would not continue to evolve in a positive direction. Many eugenicists on both sides of the Atlantic in fact spoke of degeneration, of an intellectual and physical (and thus spiritual) devolution.[148] As Nietzsche noted, the Superman was therefore needed. The Superman would be the symbol of a new form of spirituality, which sought the continued evolution of the species 'upward' by reinstituting natural selection and allowing only the best humans to breed.[149] Like many eugenicists in both the United States and Germany, Nietzschie believed that a new religious tradition would put human breeding in the foreground as a primary human virtue.[150]

Notes

1   Sections of this chapter were previously published in G.V O'Brien and A. Molinari, 'Religious metaphors as a justification for eugenic control: An historical analysis', in D. Schumm and M. Stoltzfus (eds.), *Disability in Judaism, Christianity and Islam: Sacred Texts, Historical Traditions and Social Analysis* (New York: Palgrave Macmillan, 2011), pp. 141–65. Reproduced with permission of publisher.

2   'A new force in the war on feeble-mindedness', *Survey* 29 (1913), 488.

3   'Christ was an Aryan', *Living Age* 352 (1937), 321.

4   R. Thurston, 'The Nazi war on medicine', *New Republic* 84 (4 December 1935), 100–2.

5   Klein, *Threads of Life*, pp. 39–44, 58.

6   Linnaeus quotation in R. Olby, *Origins of Mendelism* (Chicago: University of Chicago Press, 1985), p. 32.

7   Lovejoy, *The Great Chain of Being*, p. 202.

8   Chamberlain, *Foundations of the Nineteenth Century*; De Gobineau, *The Inequality of Human Races*. Also see Gould, *The Mismeasure of Man*, and Horsman, *Race and Manifest Destiny*.

9   Smith, *Minds Made Feeble*, p. 2.

10   See, for example, S. Chorover, *From Genesis to Genocide* (Cambridge, MA: M.I.T. Press, 1979), p. 41; Noël, *Intolerance*, p. 125.

11   A.E. Wiggam, *The Next Age of Man* (Indianapolis: Bobbs-Merrill Company, 1927), p. 35.

12   Hadamar, a small town located in western Germany, was the site of one of the six asylums outfitted with gas chambers as part of the T-4 euthanasia program. After this program had run its course, the facility was used for the extermination of political prisoners and other 'enemies of the Reich'.

13   E.W. Kintner (ed.), *Trial of Alfons Klein, Adolf Wahlmann, Heinrich Ruoff, Karl*

Willig, Adolf Merkle, Irmgard Huber, and Philipp Blum (the Hadamar Trial) (London: William Hodge and Company, Limited, 1949), p. 102.

14 K.M. Ludmerer, *Genetics and American Society* (Baltimore: Johns Hopkins University Press, 1972), p. 17. See also Kevles, *In the Name of Eugenics*, pp. 60–1, 68; O'Brien, 'Protecting the social body', p. 196.

15 Galton, 'Eugenics: Its definition, scope, and aims', p. 5.

16 Galton, 'Eugenics as a factor in religion', in *Essays in Eugenics*, pp. 68–70.

17 Very simply, 'perfectionism' was a doctrine which held that, through a set of spiritual and social rules, collective groups could be brought closer to God and create 'heavenly' communities on earth. These communities were especially in vogue in the mid-1800s. For more, see any of the sources for the Oneida Community listed in n. 18 below.

18 For the Oneida Community, see M.L. Carden, *Oneida: Utopian Community to Modern Corporation* (Baltimore: Johns Hopkins University Press, 1969), R.A. Parker, *A Yankee Saint* (New York: G.P. Putnam's Sons, 1935), C.N. Robertson, *Oneida Community* (Syracuse: Syracuse University Press, 1970), or S. Klaw, *Without Sin: The Life and Death of the Oneida Community* (New York: Penguin Press, 1993).

19 Wiggam, *The New Decalogue of Science*, p. 104.

20 Warthin, 'A biologic philosophy', p. 89. Not all eugenicists, however, supported framing eugenics as a new religion. For an opposing view, see R. Pearl, 'Biology and human progress', *Harper's Monthly Magazine* 172 (1935–6), 228.

21 Whitney, *The Source of Crime*, p. 4.

22 P.H. Bryce, 'Feeblemindedness and social environment', *American Journal of Public Health* 8 (1918), 656.

23 Hadden, *The Science of Eugenics and Sex Life*, p. 9.

24 Wiggam, *The New Decalogue of Science*, p. 110.

25 Ibid., p. 111.

26 A.P. Reccord, 'A perfectly normal child', *Survey* 41 (1918), 381.

27 S.Z. Batten, 'The redemption of the unfit', *American Journal of Sociology* 14 (1908), 245.

28 Burleigh, *The Third Reich*, p. 358.

29 Whitney, *The Source of Crime*, p. 16.

30 Wiggam, *The New Decalogue of Science*, pp. 110–11 (italics in original).

31 C. Rosen, *Preaching Eugenics: Religious Leaders and the American Eugenics Movement* (Oxford: Oxford University Press, 2004), p. 129.

32 Ibid., p. 111.

33 Ibid., chapter 4.

34 I. Fisher, 'Impending problems of eugenics', *Scientific Monthly* 13 (1921), 225.

35 Hooton, *Crime and the Man*, p. 398.

36 'Prizes for sermons on eugenics', *Eugenical News* 11:3 (1926), 48. See also 'Committee on Cooperation with Clergymen', *Eugenical News* 10:5 (1925), 68, and Kevles, *In the Name of Eugenics*, pp. 60–1. For more on both the prizes

for sermons and the Committee on Cooperation with Clergymen, see Rosen, *Preaching Eugenics*, chapter 4.

37 Rosen, *Preaching Eugenics*, p. 122.

38 W. Whetham and C. Whetham, *The Family and the Nation: A Study in Natural Inheritance and Social Responsibility* (London: Longmans, Green, and Co., 1909), p. 225.

39 Sumner, 'The health certificate', p. 510; see also 'Eugenics supported by the church', *Current Literature* 52 (1912), 564–6.

40 Rosen, *Preaching Eugenics*, p. 61.

41 Ibid., pp. 70–2.

42 E. Huntington and L.F. Whitney, *The Builders of America* (New York: William Morrow and Co., 1927), p. 132. See also Popenoe and Johnson, *Applied Eugenics*, p. 141. For more specific information on Catholicism and American eugenics, see Hasian, *The Rhetoric of Eugenics in Anglo-American Thought*, chapter 5.

43 'Was the doctor right?', p. 24.

44 Ibid., p. 25.

45 Kennedy, 'Euthanasia: To be or not to be', p. 16.

46 Schwartz, 'Nature's corrective principle in social evolution', p. 88.

47 Huntington and Whitney, *The Builders of America*, p. 136 (italics in original).

48 Barr, 'The prevention of mental defect, the duty of the hour', pp. 366–7.

49 K.G. Wells, 'State regulation of marriage', in *Proceedings of the National Conference of Charities and Correction* (Boston: Geo. H. Ellis, 1897), p. 305.

50 MacMurchy, 'The relation of feeble-mindedness to other social problems', in *Proceedings of the National Conference on Charities and Correction*, p. 231.

51 Ibid., p. 234.

52 Warthin, 'A biologic philosophy', p. 88.

53 L.H. Baker, *Race Improvement or Eugenics: A Little Book on a Great Subject* (New York, Dodd, Mead and Company, 1912), p. 55.

54 Ibid., pp. 55–6.

55 Mott, 'The education and custody of the imbecile', p. 175.

56 Kostir, *The Family of Sam Sixty*, p. 29 (italics in original).

57 L.A. DeVilbiss, 'Better babies contests', in *Proceedings of the First National Conference on Race Betterment* (Battle Creek, MI: Race Betterment Foundation, 1914), pp. 554–5.

58 T. Robie, 'Selective sterilization for race culture', in *A Decade of Progress in Eugenics: Scientific Papers of the Third International Congress of Eugenics* (Baltimore: Williams and Wilkens Co., 1934), p. 204.

59 See, for example, M. Storer, 'The defective delinquent girl', *Journal of Psycho-Asthenics* 19 (1914), 25–30; Wiggam, 'The rising tide of degeneracy', p. 28.

60 Gosney and Popenoe, *Sterilization for Human Betterment*, p. 40.

61 E.P. Bicknell, 'Custodial care of the adult feeble-minded', *Charities Review* 5 (November 1895–June 1896), 82.

62 R.L. Dugdale, 'Hereditary pauperism', in *Proceedings of the Conference of Charities* (Boston: A. Williams & Co., 1877), p. 84.
63 See, for example, K.B. Davis, 'Feeble-minded women in reformatory institutions', *Survey* 27 (1912), 1849–51; Fernald, 'The burden of feeble-mindedness', p. 91; MacMurchy, 'The relation of feeble-mindedness to other social problems', in *Proceedings of the National Conference on Charities and Correction*, pp. 232–3; 'The menace of the feeble-minded', p. 34; J. Weidensall, 'The mentality of the unmarried mother', in *Proceedings of the National Conference of Social Work* (Chicago: National Conference of Social Work, 1917), p. 293.
64 Rafter, *White Trash*, p. 10.
65 H.H Goddard, 'The hereditary factor in feeble-mindedness', *Institution Quarterly* 4:2 (1913), 10.
66 Interestingly, in her book *Centaurs and Amazons*, Page duBois employed the same two Greek words in her description of Pandora that Goddard used to identify his famous family. DuBois referred to Pandora as a *kalon kakon*, or a 'beautiful evil'. While Goddard had not interpreted the words in exactly this way, it certainly is a fitting representation of how eugenicists viewed women such as Deborah Kallikak, as seductive but hazardous beings. See duBois, *Centaurs and Amazons*, p. 114.
67 Goddard, *The Kallikak Family*, p. 18.
68 Dugdale, *The Jukes*, p. 15.
69 G.C. Davenport, 'Hereditary crime', p. 404.
70 See, for example, Rafter, *White Trash*, pp. 7–8.
71 Guyer, 'Sterilization', pp. 40–1.
72 Popenoe and Johnson, *Applied Eugenics*, p. 154.
73 Kline, *Building a Better Race*, p. 26.
74 Ibid., p. 121.
75 Risley, 'Is asexualization ever justifiable?', p. 97.
76 See Carlson's *The Unfit*, chapter 3.
77 Fernald, 'The burden of feeble-mindedness', p. 92.
78 Hasian, *The Rhetoric of Eugenics in Anglo-American Thought*, p. 33.
79 Smith, *Minds Made Feeble*, p. 180.
80 Stoddard, *The Revolt against Civilization*, p. 250 (italics in original).
81 H.H. Hart, 'Segregation', in *Proceedings of the First National Conference on Race Betterment* (Battle Creek, MI: Race Betterment Foundation, 1914), p. 403.
82 Fernald, 'Care of the feeble-minded', p. 390.
83 J.M. Broomall, 'The helpless classes', in *Proceedings of the Association of Medical Officers of American Institutions for Idiotic and Feeble-Minded Persons* (New York: Johnson Reprint Company Limited, 1887–95), p. 41.
84 A. Johnson, 'Children who never grow up: Some adventures among the feeble-minded', *Survey* 49 (1922–23), 310–16, 340.
85 Wolfensberger, *The Principle of Normalization in Human Services*, pp. 23–4.
86 Barr, 'The imbecile and epileptic *versus* the tax-payer and the community', p. 163.

87   A. Johnson, 'Custodial care', in *Proceedings of the National Conference of Charities and Correction* (Fort Wayne, IN: Press of Fort Wayne Printing Co., 1908), p. 336.

88   Zenderland, *Measuring Minds*, p. 200.

89   Ibid., p. 218.

90   Whetham and Whetham, *The Family and the Nation*, p. 213.

91   M.W. Barr, 'Defective children: Their needs and their rights', *International Journal of Ethics* 8 (1898), 487.

92   M.W. Barr, 'The prevention of mental defect, the duty of the hour', pp. 364–5.

93   Ibid., p. 365.

94   B.T. Sanborn, 'The care of the feeble-minded', in *Proceedings of the National Conference on Charities and Correction* (Press of Fred J. Heer, 1904), p. 405.

95   Johnson, 'Custodial care', p. 336.

96   Murdoch, 'Quarantine mental defectives', p. 66; Barr, 'Defective children', pp. 487–8.

97   A. Johnson, 'Permanent custodial care: Report of Committee on the Care of the Feeble-Minded', in *Proceedings of the National Conference on Charities and Correction* (Boston: Geo. H. Ellis, 1896), p. 216.

98   Popenoe and Johnson, *Applied Eugenics*, p. 146.

99   Mott, 'The education and custody of the imbecile', p. 174.

100 Zenderland, *Measuring Minds*, p. 177.

101 S.J. Barrows, in 'Discussion on provision for the feeble-minded', in *Proceedings of the National Conference on Charities and Correction* (Boston: Geo. H. Ellis, 1888), p. 401.

102 E.R. Johnstone, 'Committee report: Stimulating public interest in the feeble-minded', in *Proceedings of the National Conference of Charities and Correction* (Chicago: Hildmann Printing Co., 1916), p. 213.

103 Barr, 'President's annual address', p. 6.

104 Quoted in Trent, *Inventing the Feeble Mind*, p. 193.

105 Quoted in A. Cockburn, 'Beat the devil', *The Nation* (23 November 1992), 618.

106 *Buck v. Bell*, 143 Va. Ct. App., p. 318. The decision went on to note that sterilization 'in most cases relieves the patient from further confinement in the Colony [institution]', p. 319.

107 For example, see Stoddard, *The Revolt against Civilization*, p. 249n.; Wiggam, *The Next Age of Man*, p. 350.

108 Wiggam, *The Next Age of Man*, p. 352.

109 Ibid., p. 351.

110 E.A. Whitney and M.M. Shick, 'Some results of selective sterilization', in *American Association for the Study of the Feebleminded: Proceedings and Addresses of the Fifty-Fifth Annual Session* (American Association for the Study of the Feebleminded, 1931), pp. 332–3.

111 Ibid., pp. 334–5.

112 Landman, 'Race betterment by human sterilization', p. 295.

113   E.A. Whitney, 'A plea for the control of feeble-mindedness', *Eugenics* 2:5 (1929), 12.

114   T.E. Hinshaw, 'Physician's report', in *Twenty-Second Biennial Report of the State Training School, Winfield Kansas* (Topeka: Kansas State Printing Plant, 1924), p. 19.

115   Weindling, *Health, Race and German Politics*, p. 454.

116   Popenoe and Johnson, *Applied Eugenics*, p. 152.

117   Robie, 'Selective sterilization for race culture', p. 203.

118   J.B.S. Haldane, *Heredity and Politics* (New York: W.W. Norton & Company, 1938), p. 102.

119   D.M. LeBourdais, 'Purifying the human race', *North American Review* 238 (1934), 436.

120   Gosney and Popenoe, *Sterilization for Human Betterment*, p. 30.

121   Ibid., p. 33.

122   Ibid., pp. 31–2.

123   Dudziak, 'Oliver Wendell Holmes as a eugenic reformer', p. 852.

124   Lennox, 'Should they live?', p. 466.

125   McKim, *Heredity and Human Progress*, p. 188 (italics in original).

126   Huntington and Whitney, *The Builders of America*, p. 84.

127   Ibid., p. 85.

128   Pernick, *The Black Stork*, p. 6.

129   Ibid., p. 98.

130   As Fredric Wertham noted, the term 'euthanasia' was a 'misnomer' for the German program. The term refers to a 'good death', which is not at all what the victims of the Nazis experienced. See Wertham, *A Sign for Cain*, pp. 155–6.

131   Binding and Hoche, 'Permitting the destruction of unworthy life', p. 241.

132   Ibid., p. 254.

133   In order to cover up the killings, families were told that victims had died of a contagious disease or other fabricated cause.

134   Condolence letter quoted in Müller-Hill, *Murderous Science*, p. 104.

135   E. Leiser, *Nazi Cinema*, trans. G. Mander and D. Wilson (New York: Macmillan Publishing Co., Inc., 1974), p. 92.

136   Ibid., pp. 91–3.

137   See Burleigh, *Death and Deliverance*, pp. 95–6, and *The Third Reich*, pp. 383–4.

138   Wilmarth, 'Report of Committee on Feeble-Minded and Epileptic', p. 156.

139   Bancroft, 'Classification of the mentally deficient', p. 194; F.B. Kirkbride, 'The right to be well-born', *Survey* 27 (1912), 1838–9.

140   H.H. Goddard, *Feeble-Mindedness: Its Causes and Consequences* (New York: Macmillan Co., 1914), p. 558.

141   R.R. Rentoul, 'Proposed sterilization of certain mental degenerates', *American Journal of Sociology* 12 (1906), 325.

142   J. Taft, 'Supervision of the feebleminded in the community', in *Proceedings of the National Conference of Social Work* (Chicago: Rogers & Hall Co., 1918), p. 545.

143 L.J. Cole, 'Biological eugenics', *Journal of Heredity* 5 (1914), 307.
144 C. Frankel, 'The specter of eugenics', *Commentary* 57 (March 1974), 29.
145 See, for example, D. Nelkin and S.L. Gilman, 'Placing blame for devastating disease', *Social Research* 55 (1988), 368.
146 Wolfensberger, *The Principle of Normalization in Human Services*, pp. 21–4.
147 F. Nietzsche, *Thus Spoke Zarathustra*, trans. R.J. Hollingdale, reprint edn. (London: Penguin Books, 1969), p. 115.
148 Galton himself even contended that the species had been evolving backward for thousands of years. Also see E.A. Hooton's various writings on the topic of degeneration, including the books *Apes, Men and Morons, Crime and the Man,* and *The American Criminal: An Anthropological Study,* reprint edn. (New York: Greenwood Press, 1969).
149 For Nietzsche's various writings detailing human degeneration, the inherent inequality of various human groups, and the need for evolution 'upward', see *Thus Spoke Zarathustra,* pp. 41–3, 72, 104, 123–4, 228, 293–8, *Twilight of the Idols/The Antichrist,* trans. R.J. Hollingdale, reprint edn. (New York: Penguin Books, 1968), pp. 30, 55–8, 79, 85–91, 178, and *Beyond Good and Evil,* trans. W. Kaufman, reprint edn. (New York: Vintage Books, 1966), pp. 111, 201, 212–14.
150 See M.A. Mügge, 'Eugenics and the superman: A racial science, and a racial religion', *Eugenics Review* 1 (1909–10), 184–206. Also see Childs, *Modernism and Eugenics,* pp. 4–7.

6

THE OBJECT METAPHOR: THE MORON AS A POORLY FUNCTIONING HUMAN[1]

The chemical laboratory and the scientific chemist have made from the by-products of coal and petroleum, once thrown away, illuminating gas and aniline dyes of all the hues of the rainbow, benzene, gasoline and all the paraffins ... It would be still better for the country to make [something] out of life's dregs and by-products, out of lives now wasted and worse than wasted ...[2]

A principal means of diminishing the status of marginalized individuals is to objectify them; this includes referring to them as, comparing them to, or treating them as devalued inanimate objects. Another method of objectification is the development within the culture of a 'value hierarchy', wherein humans are differentially valued on the basis of their presumptive abilities, assets, or characteristics. As with the animalization of 'lower' humans on racial and philosophical hierarchies (e.g., the Great Chain of Being), the further down one falls in a hierarchy based on perceived utility or valuation, the higher the probability that one will be both objectified and subject to aversive social policies.

Those belonging to marginalized groups will often be depersonalized by being viewed not as individuals in their own right but as simply members of the group. As discussed previously, a person's master status, or primary source of identity, may be imposed upon her or him by the group in power, who will additionally define what specific roles group members may take on, as well as describe what constitutes proper or normative role behavior. Thus issues surrounding self- and other-identification are central to discussions of objectification.[3] As Lise Noël wrote,

The very meaning of alienation is that it estranges people from themselves. Adopting the image created by the oppressor, the dominated see themselves through others' eyes. Like the mentally ill, to which the term was initially applied, the alienated cease to belong to themselves.[4]

William Brennan added that through objectification people become property of others that can be manipulated at will, and even disposed of when no
longer useful.[5] They become, in other words, the property or pawns of those
who direct the labeling process. Since the ability to exert control and even
ownership are both closely related to the capacity to identify, label, or diagnose
the other, the desire to break away from this 'identification by others' has been
a primary factor in virtually all human rights movements,[6] and concerns over
objectification tend to rise during periods of raised consciousness and efforts
to expand civil rights.[7] Control over the 'other' also means that those who have
such power (or who desire to have it) can depict and display them in ways
that support a desired pejorative image of the devalued group. Photographs,
video images, and other such depictions may be specifically designed to foster
certain stereotypical qualities of the members of the group.

As noted in Chapter 2, a central element of the organism metaphor is the
presumption that the value of individuals is best gauged by the degree to which
they demonstrate qualities that are beneficial to the functioning of the whole,
or the extent to which they embrace 'appropriate' cultural values and hold
to accepted normative behavior. It is important to realize, however, that the
traits that individuals need to demonstrate in order to be fully accepted within
the community are not always 'behavioral' in nature, but are often immutable
qualities over which the individual has no control, such as race, ethnicity, or
disability status.

The fixed nature of target group classification also enhances the objectification of its members. Since they cannot change their nature or assimilate within
the majority, their master status may be made to appear as a permanent non-
malleable feature. During United States Congressional hearings on Japanese
internment, for example, a Mississippi legislator noted that there were no
appreciable differences between Japanese-Americans that corresponded to
their length of residency in the country. Even if they belonged to the third or
fourth generation of a family residing in the United States, he said, 'we cannot
trust them ... Once a Jap always a Jap. You cannot change him. You cannot
make a silk purse out of a sow's ear.'[8] Similarly, both American and Nazi
anti-Semitism held not only was that the Jew an alien within the country in
which he or she resided, but moreover that this status was permanent. Writers
frequently referred to the persistence of the 'Jewish type'. Daniel Goldhagen
noted that in Germany prior to Hitler, many who wrote on the subject
described 'the Jews' nature to be unchangeable',[9] and additionally held that
the long-standing belief that baptism could convert Jews into Christians was
erroneous, since they would always maintain their Jewish essence.[10]

A core concern of objectification is that the categorization of target group members becomes difficult when considering conditions that grade over into the 'general' population, such as race, political affiliation, and, as further discussed below, moronity. Therefore, an important goal of social control movements is the attempt to find what appears to be an accurate means of categorization. Racial anthropologists, for example, especially in Nazi Germany but elsewhere as well, spent a great deal of effort in attempting to measure the physical attributes of Jews so that they could devise a method of accurately defining members of the class. The fact that the group cannot be readily identified or diagnosed benefits those individuals and institutions that arise to classify such groups, giving them a degree of power and control. One example of this is the racial classification system that was developed in Virginia during the 1920s for the purpose of supporting laws prohibiting miscegenation.[11]

At times devalued individuals and groups may be objectified by being compared to poorly made or substandard products. Some of those who supported expanding the inspection of immigrants during the immigration restriction period in the United States (1890–1924), for example, viewed these physical and mental examinations as a form of quality control similar to what one might create in an automobile factory.[12] A pervasive view of immigrants at the time was that they were interchangeable tools of industry. While they were welcomed when low-wage work was needed for projects such as work on the railroads, their utility became marginal when such projects were completed, and they were seen as little more than excess inventory, or as 'miscellaneous human cargoes' deposited on the nation's shores.[13] Such immigrants, it was argued, did 'not form the material out of which a great nation can be built'.[14] Group members may also be viewed as being of similar value to, and thus interchangeable with, certain objects. The Nazis, for example, frequently attempted to barter with international Jewish rescue groups, trading the lives of Jews for items which they needed but were scarce during wartime.[15]

Certainly the most horrendous application of the object metaphor occurs when the marginalized group is not only treated or referred to as an inanimate object, but actually turned into one. During the Nazi regime, a cottage industry developed that was based on the collection and use of human remains for 'professional' or personal reasons. According to Evelyn Le Chêne, one Nazi physician was so taken with the craniums of two Dutch Jews that he had them made into paperweights.[16] In addition to removing the gold teeth from victims, German physicians used the brains and other body parts of 'interesting cases' for medical and anthropological study. The organs that were sent to research centers were marked 'War Material – Urgent' and 'were given top priority in transit'.[17] Not all of this 'material', however, was used for research purposes. A German anatomist described an 'anatomy guessing game' that he created for his medical students. The prizes included 'a very nice skull' and other assorted human bones.[18]

According to James Weingartner, German officials did not stand alone in collecting human remains as keepsakes of battle. United States soldiers, he noted, mutilated Japanese combatants and kept their body parts as war trophies, to the degree that it became a concern to customs officials.[19] While it is quite clear how this practice reinforces the 'person as object' metaphor, Weingartner contends that it also supports the view of the enemy as animalistic. He quotes an American general as saying that 'killing a Japanese was like killing a rattlesnake'. Therefore, Weingartner surmises, 'it was not inappropriate to preserve as a token of the fatal encounter something analogous to the reptile's rattle or skin'.[20]

The object metaphor and the moron

In speaking of the eugenic family studies, Nicole Rafter discussed the 'relentless objectification of their subjects – their insistence on turning people into things'.[21] She added that 'the family study authors turned "the real thing" – the subjects they studied – into a set of signs. By carefully selecting descriptions, using bumpkin pseudonyms, and sending covert signals to readers, the authors constructed a symbolic world'.[22] Importantly, the term 'moron', as a word that was only created shortly after the turn of the century, and roughly at the beginning of the eugenics movement, gave supporters the opportunity to invest whatever symbolic rhetoric they desired into it. This issue will be taken up again in the final chapter of this book. As is described below, a rather large collection of objects was employed to give meaning to the term 'moron', as well as to reinforce the importance of fully implementing eugenic policies.

The horticultural metaphor

Just as animal breeding was instrumental in explaining human eugenics to the lay public, plant breeding was also employed in the same way.[23] Thus children were often characterized as the 'most valuable crop' that the community could cultivate.[24] 'The human harvest', Michael Guyer noted, 'like the grain harvest is based fundamentally on heritage, and to get a better crop of boys and girls we must, as with other crops, weed out bad strains.'[25] Within this context, of course, morons and other undesirable breeders were objectified as the 'human weeds' who threatened to choke out – primarily through their rapid growth – the good crops. In the human garden a feeble-minded person was characterized as 'a social flower of no prospective bloom'.[26] Another eugenicist wrote that '[j]ust as thorns and thistles are the direct result of imperfect vegetable development, so are fools and lunatics an instance of degeneration and imperfection in human development'.[27] Unlike the care that was taken in breeding plants, one eugenicist wrote, in 'the human harvest ... we plant largely from the worst seed, and largely in the worst soil'.[28] As described in the previous chapter, Biblical verses were employed by some eugenicists to compare various sub-populations to 'good' or 'bad' seed. In addition to drawing this analogy,[29] in their book *The Builders of America* Huntington and Whitney referred to 'dysgenic' persons as 'genuine human weeds'.[30] Other eugenicists said that 'imbeciles' were 'sowing their seeds of degeneracy on a thousand hills',[31] and that '[i]t does no violence to our humanitarian ideas to take care of the present crop of undesirables on condition that they shall not act as seeds for future crops'.[32]

Beyond simply keeping down the weeds, eugenicists argued that they also needed to maintain and fertilize the good seed. In 1936 Harry Laughlin, then one of the most important supporters of eugenics in the United States, was accorded an honorary degree by the University of Heidelberg, ostensibly for his impact (especially through his support for the implementation of state sterilization laws) on the German eugenic program. In a letter wherein he acknowledged his 'deep gratitude' for the award, he noted that '[t]o me this honor will be doubly valued because it will come from a nation which for many centuries nurtured the human seed-stock which later founded my own country and thus gave basic character to our present lives and institutions'.[33]

The use of patients (especially morons, since they were 'higher-functioning') as unpaid field hands in private or asylum-run farms during the eugenic era may have reinforced the widespread employment of the horticultural metaphor. In Alexander Johnson's article entitled 'Mixed crops', for example, which was published in 1923 in the *Survey*, a major social science journal of the time, it is somewhat difficult even to tell whether the mixed crops to which the author alludes are the products of the farms or the feeble-minded boys themselves.[34]

Perhaps the most important writer to compare human and plant breeding was the famous horticulturist Luther Burbank. In his book *The Training of the Human Plant*, Burbank wrote that he had long been aware of the similarity between the development of plants and that of humans. In the fourth chapter of his book, Burbank likened child-raising to growing plants. Most of his suggestions are environmental in nature (e.g., providing sunshine, fresh air, and proper nutrition), and thus his comparisons are more euthenic than eugenic.[35] Burbank supported restrictive marriage laws for 'unfit' persons, noting that when two poisonous plants are merged, the resulting offspring is often more virulent than either parent strain.[36] He did caution, however, that we should not be too hasty in our response to the seemingly 'abnormal', saying that proper environment and care could improve 'weak' children just as they could strengthen feeble plants.[37]

The horticulture metaphor also was important within the context of the eugenic family studies, which described family 'trees' with diseased 'branches'. Elizabeth Yukins wrote:

> Goddard embellishes upon the arboreal metaphor when he describes Martin Kallikak as a 'scion' who warps the family tree by engendering this 'degenerate offshoot'. The *Oxford English Dictionary* defines the term 'scion' as a descendant or an heir, and as 'a shoot or twig'. According to Goddard's description, Martin Kallikak is a renegade scion whose actions cause the Kallikak family tree to develop a perverted outgrowth ... due to illegitimate mixing.[38]

The disease was, however, not superficial but contained within the genetic structure of the persons, or, to carry the analogy further, the roots of the tree. A superficial trimming of the diseased portion of the tree would do little long-term good, both because the disease could spread to healthy trees and because its essential nature, like that of the degenerate person, could not be changed, regardless of the care and attention given to it. Pruning, however, provided a useful eugenic metaphor where the tree represented the 'human body' or the species as a whole as opposed to an individual or family.[39]

Because of its importance in the Nazi eugenic program, a brief description of their employment of the horticultural metaphor is in order. In discussing Nazi eugenics, Burleigh wrote that '[t]otalitarian regimes are sometimes described as "gardening states", which sought to transform society by eradicating those they regarded as "alien" or "unfit", so that the "fit" might flourish'.[40] Certainly this was never truer than in Nazi Germany, where eugenic programs were under the direction of Heinrich Himmler, who had a strong interest and academic training in agriculture. Himmler's mentor, Richard Darré, the creator of the Nazi 'Blood and Soil' program, also had an important early influence on the relationship between the philosophical underpinnings of controlled human breeding and agrarian policy in Hitler's Germany. A central theme for both Darré and Himmler was that the German population could in many ways be described through agricultural analogies, and such terminology was frequently used to buttress the Nazis' eugenic programs, over which Himmler had a great deal of authority.[41]

Waste products, refuse, and objects of production

The low esteem in which eugenicists held feeble-minded persons was never clearer than in their depiction of such persons as 'an ever increasing flood of social wastage'[42] or 'refuse pieces of humanity, hardly fit to be called human beings'.[43] Of the 'feeble-minded, the epileptic and the insane', George Keene said that it was here that 'we appreciate, if ever, the existence of waste material'.[44] This 'dead weight of human waste', the birth control advocate Margaret Sanger contended, was an enormous burden to society.[45] In the following passage, Dr E.E. Southard, a pathologist and member of the board of directors of the Eugenics Record Office, holds out some hope that, as with some of the waste products of production, society may find some use for the moron;

> Coldly speaking, it becomes a question with us, what to do with these waste materials. Now the modern doctrine of efficiency in economics and other divisions of practical service is to make use of all such waste materials. I am told that we make car wheels from the refuse of cheese factories and that all the great firms are putting research men to work on the disposal of their by-products. Let us, then, look upon the feeble-minded as in some sense by-products of society.[46]

The MacMurchy quotation at the beginning of this chapter holds out the same hope that some beneficial use can be made of 'life's dregs and by-products'. The relationship between eugenics and conservationism will be further discussed below.

Referring to the 'low-grade' feeble-minded, Barr wrote that one way in which such 'waste products' could be made useful was to place them in asylums and have them perform the unskilled labor that was required to run the facility. Such a plan would not only remove such persons from society, he added, but also save taxpayers money by reducing labor costs.[47] If those who were labeled feeble-minded held any value for their productivity and occupational usefulness to society, it was in the role as a 'drudge' who would perform the low-wage menial labor that others then did not have to concern themselves with. Eugenicists discussed whether society required morons for this purpose, and whether they therefore might play some important role in the efficient running of the country. A 1916 *Literary Digest* article, for example, asked, '[w]hy not employ the feeble-minded upon public works in unskilled labor? Many mental weaklings are physically able, and manual labor would be both more healthful and more agreeable than enforced idleness'.[48] A Pennsylvania state official expressed his concern that large-scale institutionalization of morons was unwise because society would then 'also be shutting off the supply of workers to do the drudgery of the world'. 'Who', he wondered, would then 'scrub our floors and dig our ditches?'[49]

The journal *Eugenics* contributed to this discussion in 1929 with a series of brief commentaries on the topic. 'In this new and complex civilization of ours', one of these stated, 'there is no menial or necessary service which can not be done by citizens whose intelligence quotient is greater than that of the moron. In fact the so-called drudgery is being done today by machines whose operation requires skill and intelligence. More Morons? *No!*[50] Others agreed with this position, contending that more intelligent persons could perform these tasks 'more safely and efficiently', and that occupational advances made low-wage industrial workers less necessary than in the past. Huntington and Whitney felt that if society focused on measures of positive eugenics, and thereupon developed policies such as tax incentives that resulted in an increase in the birth of 'high-grade' persons, these creative and inventive individuals would naturally help to develop 'labor-saving machinery', which would further diminish the need for unskilled menial employees.[51]

Streamlining, efficiency, and eugenics

In many ways the eugenic goal of 'perfecting man' ran parallel to product development trends of the time. Christina Cogdell, in her book *Eugenic Design*, wrote that in both human and product engineering, issues such as streamlining and efficiency were invoked to support the movement to ensure that 'form followed function' when it came to both mechanical and human bodies. Both 'industrial designers and eugenicists', she contended,

> considered themselves primary agents of evolutionary progress. Assuming a role heretofore reserved to plant and animal breeders, both groups of designers rationally selected between desirable and undesirable traits to reform 'primitive', 'criminal', and 'degenerate' products and bodies into functional, 'fit' forms suitable for mass (re)production.[52]

Just as product streamlining removed anything that produced drag and detracted from the efficiency of a vehicle or product, a large-scale eugenic program would lead to the streamlining of the species, producing humans who would move through the world with as little physical, psychological, or social friction as possible. The eugenics movement reached its peak at the same time as industrial efficiency was becoming recognized as an important goal of industry. The writings of Frederick Taylor and others focused attention on the need to measure and continually improve the efficient creation of products in order to maintain a competitive advantage and enhance a business's bottom line.[53] A downside to this focus, obviously, was that it supported the objectification of workers, and especially those in the 'unskilled' labor force. The efficiency movement not only highlighted the need for competent workers, but also supported the perception that personal identification in large part related to occupational usefulness.

Some eugenicists said that anchors, weights, and brakes provided useful metaphors for describing the impact of morons on their families and the nation. As others attempted to move forward and progress, and as the nation tried to gain a competitive advantage over other countries, these individuals and other degenerates were weighing down the rest, making progress difficult and acting as 'dragnets or sheet anchors on the progress of the ship of state'.[54] Such persons were said to be a 'deplorable drag upon the wheels of progress'.[55] 'The strong and competent and moral, the free in body and in spirit', Haven Emerson wrote, 'are shackled to those whose disablements so wring our hearts that our spirits cannot push on to the higher levels of achievement.'[56] Karl Schwartz added that the feeble-minded acted as 'a drag to the car of human progress'.[57] Just as it was necessary to let off the brakes in order to 'increase the speed and efficiency of a train of cars', to 'make satisfactory social progress it is no less necessary to relieve society of its drag than it is to give it added impetus'.[58]

Cogdell wrote that the 'ability of some eugenicists to consider humans as products reveals the conceptual shift on their part to an industrial way of thinking about humanity, one that ultimately permitted the devaluation of those humans deemed less desirable by those in control'.[59] To designers and engineers of the time, she noted, product streamlining was not simply a matter of making superficial changes in the product, but took into account the entire design and production process, just as the efficient design of humans needed to consider all aspects of the individual, down to and including one's genetic structure. With both products and human beings, she added, true beauty was seen as inherent, and was closely connected to the efficiency of the machine or body. Just as physical attractiveness and 'fitness' were related in the minds of eugenicists, engineers believed that the aesthetic appeal of a streamlined product was an obvious outgrowth of its efficient design.[60] Anti-immigration supporters and eugenicists frequently decried the unkempt look and 'crooked faces' of lower-class non-Nordic immigrants, and felt that these inefficient bodies were rapidly diminishing the aesthetic figure of 'native' Americans, as well as being a manifestation of underlying degeneration.[61]

The 'conservation' of the species was viewed by eugenicists as similar to efficiency and streamlining. Just as the latter two terms were employed as mechanistic metaphors to describe the development of a better human product, the former term carried the theme of natural conservation to the human realm. 'Is there a demand for conservation of human resources', one eugenicist asked, 'while we are exercising our souls about timber, water-power, coal, and natural gas?'[62] Similarly, in his 1914 address at the First National Conference on Race Betterment, Leon Cole remarked:

[W]e are saying that the material benefits of our forests, our minerals, and our water power must be conserved for the benefit of all the people, and not reaped now to enrich a few individuals and to be passed on only to their families. Shall we have less foresight in the heritage of defectives and cripples that we pass on to the next and future generations? Is not the social reformer who does not take this into consideration spending all his thought on bettering the present generation, just as exhausting our national resources might enrich this generation but pauperize the next?[63]

If morons and other undesirable groups were a form of societal 'pollution', or if their mingling with persons of 'good' germ plasm infected and thus depleted this important resource, the community had as much right to pass social policies designed to bring this under control as any other deleterious or toxic consequence of manufacturing. L. Pierce Clark saw morons in just this way, writing in the *Survey* in 1912 that they were a 'pitiable by-product in the evolution of the human race'.[64]

Conservation arguments in support of eugenic control have been readily accepted at times of scarce or depleted resources, as when rationing is a necessity during wartime. There is a strong temptation in such periods 'to adopt a narrowly materialistic perspective for the establishment of priorities and to seek savings through short cuts at the expense of those who were weak and less able to defend themselves'.[65] Certainly conservation-based rhetoric was also favored by those advocates of eugenics who, like Theodore Roosevelt, were in fact conservationists. Probably the most important of these was Madison Grant. Grant was a zoologist and a leading voice within the movement during its later period.[66] As the biographer Jonathan Spiro said of Grant, 'as a conservationist he found that eugenics harmonized with his concurrent development of wildlife management'.[67] According to this social Darwinistic line of reasoning, strong species were created when predators were able to 'cull the herd', a process which was no longer allowed in regard to the human species.

Within the context of conservation, it was the immortal germ plasm that was the object of concern.[68] Eugenic rhetoric often objectified individuals by portraying them as carriers, vehicles, or vessels that stored and transmitted 'good' or 'bad' germ plasm.[69] If a sound body and mind were 'the most priceless of human possessions', then it followed that the most important human 'commodity' was the germ plasm that created them.[70] Aldred Scott Warthin, presaging Nazi rhetoric, said that there 'can be no real medicine that does not consider the germ plasm … [and] the hereditary constitution of the individual as the important thing'.[71]

Conservation of preferred germ plasm and the perception of the moron as a source of pollution came together in the 'stream' metaphor that ran throughout much eugenic writing. As noted in Chapter 2, eugenicists contended that defective individuals threatened the integrity of the water supply that is the life source of the species, the germ plasm. As Cogdell noted, a number of them employed this metaphor, comparing their program to water conservation. Many of the sermons that preachers entered for the eugenic competition, she wrote, included the image of the 'unpolluted blood stream' contrasted with those streams that were becoming stagnant from the 'putrefaction of criminal strains' and the 'currents and eddies of diseased mind or enfeebled intellect'.[72]

The diminished value of the moron

In these images of the moron as a weed choking beautiful flowers, a brake slowing the train of progress, a worthless by-product of human evolution, an unessential menial laborer, or a defective and inefficient product of manufacturing, the message was clear: feeble-minded persons were of no appreciable value to the community. They were 'without value to themselves or to the rest of the world'.[73] If, as Galton stated, 'the parents of noteworthy children' were 'the contributors of ... valuable assets to the national wealth', the parents of defective and dependent children were liabilities for which everyone paid a heavy cost.[74]

In the American eugenic literature there is much discussion of various groups as assets or liabilities to the nation. Edward East, for example, wrote that some children 'are not worth 5,000 brass farthings – they are liabilities, not assets; others are worth golden millions. If prosperity is to be promoted, the assets should be increased and the liabilities reduced'.[75] Lothrop Stoddard fused the conservationist language described above with 'value' rhetoric:

> In the same way that some scientists survey our natural resources and map out our material wealth in ore deposits, oil fields and agricultural soils, other scientists are examining our human resources and are analyzing our human wealth ... it is safe to say that the time is not far distant when we shall be able to draw up some sort of rough balance sheet of our human assets and liabilities.[76]

Referring to the eugenically 'fit', he added that the 'rich stores of human treasure' could be perceived as 'assets to offset our unfortunately numerous human liabilities'.[77] The Jukes, another article proclaimed, would be looked upon by a future society as 'an unnecessary luxury' that it could ill afford to maintain.[78]

As discussed in Chapter 4, the lives of feeble-minded persons and soldiers were often compared for the purpose of comparing what were typically viewed as the most valueless and valuable lives. During World War I an American writer decried the fact that '[w]hile the perfect specimens of our manhood are off at the front, getting maimed or killed, the feebleminded are at home living on the efforts of other people and procreating ever-increasing numbers of their own kind'.[79] In their 1920 book that presaged the Nazi euthanasia program, Binding and Hoche wrote as follows;

> Reflect simultaneously on a battlefield strewn with thousands of dead youths, or a mine in which methane gas has trapped hundreds of energetic workers; compare this with our mental hospitals, with their caring for their living inmates. One will be deeply shaken by the strident clash between the sacrifice of the finest flower of humanity in its full measure on the one side, and by the meticulous care shown to existences which are not just absolutely worthless but even of negative value, on the other.[80]

The differential value of various persons was clearly spelled out by Charles Davenport in his presidential address to the Third International Congress of Eugenics:

> Eugenics is not interested in death rates any more than it is in birth rates. It is interested only in quality. One may even view with satisfaction the high death rate in an institution for low grade feeble-minded, while one regards as a natural disaster the loss of a bold and successful aviator, or even the infant child of exceptional parents.[81]

A pervasive theme in discussions about infanticide over the past century is that, because of their relative value, the killing of a 'defective' infant is a lesser crime – if indeed it constitutes a crime at all – than the killing of a non-disabled infant. In regard to the previously discussed Bollinger baby case, for example, the coroner 'had indicated that unless a post-mortem proved the child, if its life had been saved by an operation, would have been a mental defective, Dr. Haiselden, chief of the hospital staff, might be tried for criminal negligence for his refusal to intervene, even though with the parents consent'.[82] In other words, what was considered murder if the child was diagnosed as non-disabled was judged to be an excusable 'mercy killing' if a disability diagnosis could be made.

Eugenics and the objectification of women

For many eugenicists in the United States, the value of women especially was directly related to both their willingness to bear children and their eugenic 'fitness'. As described in the previous chapter, females who were classified as morons or as otherwise hereditarily defective were generally identified as sexually immoral and incapable of controlling their base desires. Conversely, for a woman with 'valuable traits which she has inherited and which she can pass on to offspring, the disposition to evade this obligation' was counted as a 'manifest racial delinquency'.[83] As Elizabeth Yukins wrote, to eugenicists, 'a woman's body promised either the continuing progression of genealogical, and thus national, development, or the insidious threat of moral pathology and biological determination'.[84] Wendy Kline similarly noted that '[t]he eugenic construction of womanhood was double-edged: it contained the potential not only for racial progress but also for racial destruction'.[85]

Some eugenicists held a conservative view that supported traditional gender roles, and derided women for desiring to attend college or seeking a career as well as for waiting to marry and have children, thus contributing to race suicide.[86] Advocates of positive eugenics who considered themselves liberals, progressives, or reformers, however, needed to reconcile their support of the 'new woman' with the eugenic demand that unmarried women focus on marriage, and that married women direct their energies to child-bearing and child-rearing. Theodore Roosevelt said that women could have their cake and eat it too. He suggested that they begin their family when still young and should have many children, and that then they could work or engage in philanthropic activities when the children grew. A career, he felt, was fine so long as it was a supplement to rather than a substitute for the woman's natural role as mother.[87] Many eugenicists felt that women would voluntarily choose motherhood if it was accorded the importance it deserved. According to Kline, the 'mother of tomorrow' was, as envisioned by many eugenicists, an empowered figure, who 'controlled the racial makeup of future generations'.[88] If indeed child-bearing was viewed as a form of efficient production, women's maternal instinct could possibly – if properly framed – be considered a form of industrial activity where they themselves would have a great deal of importance in developing the most proficient means of bearing and caring for a child.

As noted in previous chapters, the issue of objectification is particularly important given the relationship of the eugenics movement to the birth control movement, especially since the latter was gaining momentum during the period in which the eugenics movement reached its apex. Since Margaret Sanger is the primary symbol of the birth control movement in the United States, her role vis-à-vis eugenics is especially instructive.[89] Sanger attempted to gain support from leading eugenicists for the birth control movement, but most of these leaders held her at arm's length. While there was general agreement between eugenicists and Sanger about negative eugenics and especially the control of those labeled as morons,[90] they disagreed in important ways when it came to positive eugenics. Most advocates of eugenics in the United States believed that the widespread dissemination of birth control information would have a dysgenic impact on society, as those who would be most apt to restrict their births would be middle- and upper-class families. They held that morons and their ilk had little capacity for such foresight. This, they felt, would support race suicide and the differential birth rate. Sanger, however, believed that all women needed to be in control of their procreation and the spacing of their children,[91] and that small families were beneficial to both the families themselves as well as an increasingly over-populated world.[92] While some leading eugenicists came around to supporting birth control late in the movement, most remained wary.

Nazi ideology should again be briefly discussed here, since the Nazis made the objectification of women a core feature of their racial philosophy.[93] Condemning the drop in the national birth rate over the first third of the century, they attempted to counteract this by launching a vigorous campaign to increase births. Declaring that 'the nation's stock of ovaries [was] a national resource and property of the German state'[94] or a central component of 'the biological capitol of the *Volk*',[95] Nazi propaganda both glorified German mothers and at the same time controlled, manipulated, and objectified them. Fertile Aryan women were frequently portrayed as the female equivalent of soldiers for the Reich, and numerous financial incentives (reduced home loans) and symbolic incentives (preferred seating on trains) were provided to those women who had large families.[96] Females from conquered territories who had 'Aryan' features, moreover, were often taken into custody to serve as 'breeders' for the Reich.[97]

The moron as an object of research or observation

One valued societal role that intellectually disabled persons have traditionally filled is the completely passive function of a research object or subject of a cautionary tale. According to Bird Baldwin,

> mentally defective children offer excellent material for psychological investigation, since they are a more or less isolated group with quite definitive boundaries and are dependent on others. They may be observed continuously during their lifetime, they are incapable of being stimulated or enthused by artificial reactions, they are not easily embarrassed or self-conscious.[98]

Therefore, he continued, they provide 'the best material at present available for the study of human heredity'.[99]

As described in Chapter 3, there is a long history of persons with mental disabilities being exploited for exhibitionary and commercial purposes. Charging visitors to gawk at and tease asylum residents, eugenic-era displays of disabled persons at world's fairs, and the employment of persons with microcephaly and other disabilities in freak shows and other forms of exhibition have served both to fascinate curious viewers who were interested in the nature of human differences and to justify measures of social control.[100]

That feeble-minded persons were viewed as objects of study during the eugenic era is clearly indicated by their frequent use as research subjects, especially, as noted above, within the context of the eugenic family studies. For eugenicists, the study of feeble-mindedness was not only a way of understanding the condition and its causes, but a path to the greater goal of eliminating feeble-mindedness from the population, not through cure but through methods of eugenic control. Those family members who were interviewed within the course of the family students were unwitting accomplices in this effort,[101] as were, according to English, those asylum inmates who were asked to volunteer to assist in typing field workers' notes.[102] Leon Cole admitted that the purpose of studying morons was not to find ways to change or cure them, since this was impossible. Speaking of such persons, he stated that we could '[m]edically inspect the earthworms in our gardens if we like, but earthworms they will be to the end of time'.[103]

Within the family studies particularly, photographs were often employed for the purpose of furthering the objectification of their subjects. As a number of authors have noted, even before the eugenic era photographs, drawings and other visual depictions had come to play an important role in the medical and psychiatric description of not only diseases but also the persons impacted by them.[104] Such photographs were utilized not simply to share diagnostic facts, however, but also to put forth a particular image of the patient or subject for ideological or even political purposes. In her book *Picture Imperfect*, Ann Maxwell discusses the various ways in which photographs and other images were utilized to further the cause of eugenics.[105] The use of 'mug shots', she notes, highlighted the supposed criminalistic nature of the members of family studies,[106] and the photographs were a means of demonstrating to viewers the wide range of humankind, and the vast differences between the best and worst specimens of the species. As Brave and Sylva wrote, '[t]he cause of eugenics was in part propelled by the visual aversion to "the unfit"'.[107] In his book *The Borderland of Imbecility*, Mark Jackson provides an insightful description of the use of photographs in Great Britain during the eugenic era to foster a desired image of feeble-mindedness:

> [V]isual images served to establish the feeble-minded in particular as a distinct and enduring sub-class in society. Photographs of the physical stigmata of deficiency rendered the feeble-minded visible, thereby facilitating the identification, surveillance, and control of a previously hidden but deviant section of the population.[108]

Those who created and disseminated photographs that denigrated their subjects could (especially when these subjects were institutional residents) pose and dress them in particular ways, use lighting, focus, and other photographic 'trickery' to enhance specific physical aspects of the persons and create a setting that supported various eugenic perspectives.[109] A particular example of the latter were photos and films commissioned by the Third Reich designed to lend support for their euthanasia program. As Burleigh noted, the most grotesque asylum patients (heads shaved and dressed alike to remove any semblance of individuality) were set against the exterior of their spacious, 'opulent' asylum. The not-so-veiled message was that in a time of war and sacrifice such persons were cared for by the state in an extravagant manner.[110]

In his book *The Black Stork* Martin Pernick provides an interesting overview of the presentation of eugenic ideals within early films in the United States. According to Pernick and as mentioned in Chapter 5 above, movies such as *The Black Stork*, a film based on the Bollinger baby infanticide case, came under pressure because of their 'aesthetic content', and often were banned because of their presentation of uncomfortable topics. Some critics opposed such films because of the possibility of 'maternal impressions', as discussed in Chapter 3.[111]

Controversy has surrounded claims, first introduced by Steven Jay Gould in his ground-breaking *The Mismeasure of Man*, that some of the photographs in the Kallikak study were purposefully retouched to make the subjects appear more sinister.[112] Whether or not these claims are true, as noted in Chapter 3, the photos of toothless hillbillies and ramshackle huts in the accounts of many of the family studies not only animalized their subjects but fostered an objectivist framing that reinforced the contentions of supporters of eugenics.

The financial cost of moronity

The perception that morons and other 'defectives' were a drain on the nation's fiscal resources often went hand in glove with arguments of race suicide and differential population growth, and supported the belief that an individual's value to society could be best gauged by whether he or she constituted a 'credit' or 'debit' to the community purse. Eugenicists generally assumed that welfare expenditures would naturally increase in conjunction with the growth in the feeble-minded population. As Malthus first discussed, this would presumably result in an increased burden on the middle and upper classes, the members of which would then face financial pressure to reduce the size of their own families. 'Feeble-mindedness in the race', Leon Whitney wrote, 'affects all of us, since we have to spend vast sums in taking care of the lower grades of

our feeble-minded people, with the realization that the thousands of them who
are free in our population, and are reproducing, will necessitate our spending
more and more.'[113]

Many eugenicists felt that even those who refused to endorse their proposals because of ethical or religious concerns would eventually turn to them
because of fiscal necessity. Some proposed increasing the amount that was
spent on research and on measures of primary prevention as opposed to the
warehousing and treatment of feeble-minded, insane, and other disabled
persons:

> If only one-half of one per cent. of the 30 million dollars annually spent on hos-
> pitals, 20 millions on insane asylums, 20 millions for almshouses, 13 millions on
> prisons, and 5 millions on the feeble-minded, deaf and blind were spent on the
> study of the bad germ-plasm that makes necessary the annual expenditure of
> nearly 100 millions in the care of its produce, we might hope to learn just how it
> is being reproduced and the best way to diminish its further spread.[114]

Others praised measures such as sterilization as money-saving measures:

> It would have cost but $150.00 to have sterilized the original [Juke] couples, to
> cut off the seemingly endless social sores resulting wherever members of these
> families have settled. Yet the actual cost in relief alone of only one of these fami-
> lies was estimated at over $2,000,000.00 in 1916, as there were at that time 2,000
> members of that socially unworthy clan. We have no idea what the cost may have
> risen to now and there are many such clans in our civilized society.[115]

While such economic arguments could be countered by the assertion that
a price tag should not be placed on human beings, pragmatic eugenicists realized that they could strike a responsive chord with the public by focusing on
the specter of the rapidly increasing tax burden which would be required to
support this expanding horde of defectives.[116] Whitney, for example, argued
that the tax burden could be decreased by 65 percent or more if the hereditarily unfit members of society were eliminated,[117] and many eugenicists would
have agreed with Kempton that 'every feeble-minded birth eliminated is
at least a financial gain'.[118] Even if taxes were not reduced through eugenic
programs, the money could at least be spent more wisely than on supporting
'burdensome' lives. This presumption again relates to the efficiency argument.
Margaret Sanger wrote that much better things could be done with tax money
if it was not used for the 'care and segregation of men, women, and children
who should never have been born'. This money, she continued, 'should be
available for human development, [and] for scientific, artistic and philosophic
research'.[119] C.C. Little, the President of the University of Michigan and
President of the Third Race Betterment Conference, suggested that if certain

philanthropists or groups insisted that the government not restrict the reproduction rights of 'unfit' persons, these parties should be willing to support 'the
total expense of the care of the permanent defectives' that would result from
such a hands-off policy.[120]

A great deal of eugenic propaganda was designed specifically to bring home
to the general public this impression that the targets of the movement were
an enormous tax burden. A traveling exhibit, for example, created under the
auspices of the American Eugenics Society, demonstrated the presumed cost
of degeneracy. Brought to state fairs and other large public gatherings, this
exhibit included

> a large board upon which lights flash at various intervals dramatizing national
> statistics of eugenical importance ... When another light flashes every seven
> minutes, a person is admitted to some state institution ... Data under one of the
> other lights are of importance to the tax payer: 'Every thirty-one seconds, state
> tax payers paid $100 for maintenance ... of insane, feeble-minded, epileptic,
> blind and deaf in state insititutions only, in 1927'.[121]

It is both ironic and instructive that during the Great Depression, when
economic justifications for control would have seemed to be the most applic-
able, the menace of the feeble-minded was actually diminishing in the United
States. This highlights the fact that, while marginalized populations, especially
those that can be framed as social parasites, may be more vulnerable to control
measures during tough economic times, one cannot assume a simplistic causal
relationship between the public response to such 'burdensome' populations
and the state of the economy.

While the financial burden posed by the feeble-minded and other 'degenerates' was an important element in the rhetoric of American eugenicists during
the first quarter of the century, it was even more significant in Nazi Germany.[122]
Nazi ideology exploited the dire financial position of middle-class Germans to
support the Nazis' programs of negative eugenics. Even euthanasia was referred
to by some members of the government as one of many 'economic planning'
measures.[123] Nazi officials frequently cited the amount of tax money that was
'wasted' on valueless lives, especially during the war, when money needed to
be utilized for supporting the military.[124] Incredibly, even German textbooks
included mathematical problems that required students to calculate how much
money certain dependent persons cost the state, and how many 'fit' middle-
class families could be provided with housing for the same outlay.[125] As the T-4
euthanasia program was implemented, the Nazis calculated the presumptive
savings. Discussing the 'bizarre' statistics that were found at Hartheim, one of
the six T-4 institutions, Henry Friedlander wrote that these calculations

provided an exact account of future monies saved by killing the disabled. The T-4 statistician figured that 70,273 'disinfections' saved the German Reich 885,439,980 reichsmarks over a period of ten years. Computing future savings of food, he argued that 70,273 murdered patients, for instance, saved Germany 13,492,440 kilograms of meat and sausage – a macabre utilitarianism designed to rationalize the eugenic and racial ideology that created the killing centers.[126]

Incentivizing 'normalcy'

The financial incentives proposed by some eugenicists were closely related to the perception of various groups as assets or liabilities within society. These proposals sought to restructure differential fecundity by offering financial rewards to 'fit' parents in order to encourage them to increase the number of children they had. McDougall, for example, floated the suggestion that race suicide might be countered by restructuring salaries such that employees would earn more money according to the number of children they had,[127] a recommendation that Paul Popenoe described as the 'Proportional Family Wage'.[128] Lothrop Stoddard responded to recommendations such as this by noting that these programs could have dysgenic results, since it would primarily be the low-wage – and presumably less intelligent – workers who would be stimulated by the plan. 'Only where the racial superiority of the couples in question is clearly apparent', he wrote, 'should such subsidies be granted.'[129]

Other eugenicists recommended financial incentives targeted specifically at 'unfit' groups. Under these proposals, however, recipients would get money not for having children, but for becoming sterilized. In his 1937 article 'Utopia by sterilization', H.L. Menchen suggested that the United States government pay $1,000 to all Americans who were not desirable parents upon their voluntary sterilization. Even better, he noted, philanthropists could offer up the money, relieving the taxpayer of the cost. 'Ten or fifteen million dollars', he contended, 'would be enough to rescue the whole of Arkansas' from degeneracy.[130] The cost was low, he added, 'immensely cheaper than supporting an ever-increasing herd of morons for all eternity'.[131] Interestingly, Menchen noted that his suggestion related only to the sterilization of males. Since the operation was of a more serious nature in females, he felt that they should not be induced to go through with it.[132]

Leon Whitney believed that money was not necessary. If morons were given the opportunity to choose between purchasing luxury items and spending money to raise children, he wrote, they would agree to voluntary sterilization. 'Mr. Moron', he said,

here you see a squalling baby who will get you up nights, and here you see nice long evenings in the poolroom – which will *you* choose? A Sears-Roebuck catalogue offers a thousand choices between a baby and something else that looks pretty tempting. Which will the morons choose? If you think they will choose more than one or two babies, then you don't know morons.[133]

Discussion

A principal goal of eugenic writing in the United States was to dehumanize the targets of eugenic policies through the various modes of objectification described above. Within the context of these writings, 'feeble-minded' persons became faceless stereotypes, no more deserving of individual attention than any other denigrated minority group. As Deutsch wrote, 'the underlying ideological assumption [to eugenics] was that so-called degenerates, unlike respectable people, lacked individuality'.[134] This mode of framing of persons with intellectual disabilities was not confined to the eugenic era, and a particularly graphic recent example was described by Burton Blatt:

> During my visit to the above institution, I was told about the development of a new research center on the institutional grounds. The assistant superintendent mentioned to me that the 'material' for the research center would come from the institution and this center would require the addition of approximately 30 or 40 'items' … patients are called 'material' and personnel are called 'items'. It was so difficult to believe that this assistant superintendent was not either 'pulling my leg' or using some idiosyncratic jargon that, during my subsequent visits to dormitories in that institution, I asked the attending physician 'how many "items" do you have in this building? How much "material" do you have?' To my amazement, they knew exactly what I was asking for and gave me the numbers immediately.[135]

One might assume that some of the psychological benefits that derive from objectification in wartime, national economic distress, natural catastrophe, or similar situations, described by Keen and others, have relevance in regard to the care and treatment of persons with intellectual disabilities. For example, in facilities where there are high death rates (from infectious disease, poor treatment, or abuse), it may be psychologically beneficial for workers to find ways to disassociate themselves from residents. The various elements of institutional life (denial of unique hobbies, employment, and activities, uniform schedules, food, living conditions, etc.) not only have proven beneficial in making life easier for workers and administrators, but serve to covertly allow residents to be viewed in a homogenous manner.

If the unique attributes of institutionalized residents have been historically diminished through the trappings of congregate care, it is even more true that media representations of persons with intellectual disabilities served, especially during the eugenic era, to support a desired, and largely negative, perception of the 'moron'. Discussions of moronity to which the general public was privy came almost exclusively from acknowledged experts in the field, the vast majority of whom supported eugenic policies. Presumably scientific studies that painted the feeble-minded segment of the population with a broad brush, such as those of the Kallikaks and 'Tribe of Ishmael', came to represent to the mass of the population who these groups were and the threat they posed.

The issue of 'group utility' was also an important factor in the objectification of eugenic targets. Utilitarian questions about whether the presence of feeble-minded and other 'unfit' persons within the community might be beneficial in certain ways arose frequently. Normally, as one might expect, the answer was a resounding 'no'. It should be noted, however, that utility was a much more important aspect of German eugenics under the Nazis. Here life or death itself was frequently contingent on one's ability to perform tasks that were important for the state.[136]

To return to the issue of identification by the self versus identification by others, discussed in the introduction to this chapter, those labeled as morons were identified during the period not only by others, but by others who had a vested interest in their continued control. While the eugenic alarm era in the United States waned during the 1930s, and sterilizations and forced institutionalizations several decades later, it might be argued that the conditions for large-scale control of such persons remained so long as their identity was largely fashioned by others whose interests were inimical to their own.

Notes

1 Sections of this chapter were originally published in the author's 'Anchors on the ship of progress and weeds in the human garden: Objectivist rhetoric in American eugenic writings', *Disability Studies Quarterly* 31:3 (2011), www.dsq-sds.org, accessed August 2011.

2 Helen MacMurchy, quoted in Murdoch, 'Quarantine mental defectives', p. 66.

3 Noël, *Intolerance*, p. 52 (italics in original).

4 Ibid., p. 79.

5 Brennan, *Dehumanizing the Vulnerable*, p. 127.

6 P. Freire, *Pedagogy of the Oppressed*, As Freire notes, those who seek to control others also inadvertently force a label onto themselves (as oppressors, owners, etc.) and thus also limit the range of their own actions and identity, thereupon thwarting their own potential for growth.

7 As witnessed, for example, by discussions related to the objectification of females through pornography during the women's rights movement of the 1960s and 1970s.

8   Statement of Congressman Rankin, *Congressional Record* (Washington, DC: U.S. Government Printing Office, 18 February 1942), p. 1419. Also see *Congressional Record* (26 February 1942), p. 1682.

9   D.J. Goldhagen, *Hitler's Willing Executioners: Ordinary Germans and the Holocaust* (New York: Alfred A. Knopf, 1996), p. 66.

10 Ibid., p. 68.

11 Plecker, 'Virginia's effort to preserve racial integrity', in *A Decade of Progress in Eugenics*, pp. 105–12. Also see Black, *War against the Weak*, chapter 9, and Newbeck, *Virginia hasn't Always been for Lovers*.

12 A.M. Kraut, *Silent Travelers: Germs, Genes and the 'Immigrant Menace'* (New York: Basic Books, 1994), p. 63.

13 'Immigration checks the native birth rate', *World's Work* 46 (1923), 122.

14 'The plea for immigrants a plea for inefficiency', *World's Work* 46 (1923), 122.

15 H. Höhne, *The Order of the Death's Head*, trans. R. Barry (New York: Ballantine Books, 1969), p. 636.

16 E. Le Chêne, *Mauthausen: The History of a Death Camp* (London: Methuen & Co. Ltd., 1971), p. 88; See also Wertham, *A Sign for Cain*, pp. 145–6.

17 Müller-Hill, *Murderous Science*, p. 72.

18 Aly, Chroust, and Pross, *Cleansing the Fatherland*, p. 144.

19 J. Weingartner, 'War against subhumans: Comparisons between the German war against the Soviet Union and the American war against Japan, 1941–1945', *Historian* 58 (1996), 571.

20 Ibid.

21 Rafter, *White Trash*, p. 24.

22 Ibid., p. 26.

23 See R. Brave and K. Sylva, 'Exhibiting eugenics: Response and resistance to a hidden history', *Public Historian* 29:3 (2007), 33–51.

24 Powlison, 'Behold a sower went forth to sow', p. 5. Also see Whitney's 'A plea for the control of feeble-mindedness', p. 12.

25 Guyer, 'Sterilization', p. 34.

26 H.G. Hardt, 'Care of feeble-minded women', *Institution Quarterly* 3:1 (1912), 180.

27 Keene, 'The genesis of the defective', p. 409. Also see Spiro's *Defending the Master Race*, p. 126, where he quotes Ernst Haeckel, an early German eugenic supporter, as comparing the poisoning of weeds to the killing of 'unfit specimens of humanity'.

28 A. Blount, 'Eugenics in relation to birth control', *Birth Control Review* 2:1 (1918), 7.

29 Huntington and Whitney, *The Builders of America*, p. 80.

30 Ibid., p. 75.

31 Quoted in Larson, *Sex, Race and Science*, p. 117.

32 Fisher, 'Impending problems of eugenics', p. 229.

33 Letter from H.H. Laughlin to Dr C. Schneider, dated 28 May 1936. In the last

paragraph of the letter Laughlin expressed regret that he was unable to attend the ceremony where he was to receive the honor.

34 A. Johnson, 'Mixed crops: Some more adventures among the feeble-minded', *Survey* 49 (1922–23), 439–44, 465–6.

35 L. Burbank, *The Training of the Human Plant* (New York: Century Co., 1907), pp. 30–44.

36 Ibid., pp. 58–9.

37 Ibid., pp. 53–5.

38 Yukins, 'Feeble-minded white women', p. 179.

39 For a visual image of the tree metaphor within the context of the Nazi eugenic program, see G. Bock, 'Nazi sterilization and reproductive policies', in *Deadly Medicine: Creating the Master Race* (Washington, DC: United States Holocaust Memorial Museum, 2004), p. 65.

40 Burleigh, *The Third Reich*, p. 344.

41 See, for example, Höhne, *The Order of the Death's Head*, pp. 39–44, 59; Weindling, *Health, Race and German Politics*, pp. 474–8.

42 Guyer, 'Sterilization', p. 34.

43 Barrows, in 'Discussion on provision for the feeble-minded', p. 402; also see p. 396.

44 Keene, 'The genesis of the defective', p. 413.

45 Sanger, *The Pivot of Civilization*, p. 112.

46 E.E. Southard, 'The feeble-minded as subjects of research in efficiency', in *Proceedings of the National Conference on Charities and Correction* (Chicago: Hildemann Printing Co., 1915), p. 316.

47 Barr, 'The imbecile and epileptic *versus* the tax-payer and the community', p. 165.

48 'Service from imbeciles', p. 554; Also see Humphrey, 'Men and half-men', p. 284.

49 Quoted in Sanville, 'Social legislation in the Keystone State', p. 670.

50 W.S. Anderson, in 'Does the world need more morons?', *Eugenics* 2:4 (1929), 20.

51 Huntington and Whitney, *The Builders of America*, p. 292. See also Armstrong, 'The moron menace', p. 53; Popenoe and Johnson, *Applied Eugenics*, p. 136; E.A. Whitney, 'A hunt for society's danger spot', *Eugenics* 1:1 (1928), 30. In Nazi Germany, feeble-minded persons and others with 'hereditary' disabilities were valued largely on the basis of their perceived usefulness to the state. In cases where they could be put to good use, they might be sterilized but kept alive, at least until they were no longer productive; see Burleigh, *The Third Reich*, pp. 392, 401, and G. Ziemer, *Education for Death: The Making of the Nazi* (London: Oxford University Press, 1941), p. 77.

52 C. Cogdell, *Eugenic Design: Streamlining America in the 1930s* (Philadelphia: University of Pennsylvania Press, 2004), p. 50; also see pp. 80–1.

53 See, for example, F.W. Taylor, *Scientific Management*, reprint edn. (New York: Harper & Brothers, 1947).

54 'Birth control is peril to race, says Osborn', *New York Times* (23 August 1932), 16.

55 Lyons, 'Ungraded parents', p. 340.

56 H. Emerson, 'Eugenics in relation to medicine', *Journal of Heredity* 30 (1939), 554.

57 Schwartz, 'Nature's corrective principle in social evolution', p. 74.

58 Ibid., p. 76. The image of the 'moron' and other devalued persons as burdens on society was, as one might assume, extensively employed in Nazi Germany to support eugenic goals. See, for example, Proctor, *Racial Hygiene*, figure 37; W.W. Peter, 'Germany's sterilization program', *American Journal of Public Health* 24 (1934), 190; Harrington, 'Metaphoric connections', p. 374; Burleigh, *The Third Reich*, p. 381.

59 Cogdell, *Eugenic Design*, p. 82.

60 Ibid., p. 53.

61 Nies, *Eugenic Fantasies*, p. 32.

62 'Husbanding the nation's manhood', *World's Work* 20 (1910), 13470.

63 Cole, 'The relation of philanthropy and medicine to race betterment', p. 504. See the similar statement in his 'Biological eugenics', p. 309.

64 L.P. Clark, 'Idiocy and laboratory research', *Survey* 27 (1912), 1860.

65 J. Noakes and G. Pridham (eds), *Nazism 1919–1945: A History in Documents and Eyewitness Accounts*, vol. II: *Foreign Policy, War and Racial Extermination* (New York: Schocken Books, 1988), p. 1001.

66 For Grant's eugenic writings, which focused heavily on race suicide fears, see his *The Passing of the Great Race: Or, the Racial Basis of European History* (New York: Charles Scribner's Sons, 1916), and *The Conquest of a Continent* (New York: Charles Scribner's Sons, 1933).

67 Spiro, *Defending the Master Race*, p. 134; also see p. 236.

68 For eugenicists' discussion of the 'immortal germ plasm', see ibid., pp. 134–5.

69 I. Fisher, 'Public health as a social movement', in *Proceedings of the National Conference of Social Work* (Chicago: National Conference of Social Work, 1917), pp. 183–93.

70 Quoted in Hasian, *The Rhetoric of Eugenics in Anglo-American Thought*, p. 44.

71 Warthin, 'A biologic philosophy', p. 87.

72 Quoted in Cogdell, *Eugenic Design*, pp. 55–6.

73 H.S. Jennings, *The Biological Basis of Human Nature* (New York: W.W. Norton & Company, Inc., 1930), p. 226.

74 Galton, 'Eugenics: Its definition, scope, and aims', p. 5. Also see 'The future of America', p. 530.

75 E.M. East, *Heredity and Human Affairs* (New York: Charles Scribner's Sons, 1927), p. 251.

76 Lothrop Stoddard, 'Worthwhile Americans', *Saturday Evening Post* 197 (17 January 1925), 23.

77 Ibid., 150.

78 'The Jukes in 1915', *Journal of Heredity* 7 (1916), 473.

79 C.B. Thompson, 'Conservation of minds' (letter to the editor), *Survey* 38 (1917), 362.

80 Binding and Hoche, 'Permitting the destruction of unworthy life', p. 246. This relationship was often noted in Nazi eugenic writings. The director of an asylum in the Third Reich where large numbers of disabled children were starved to death, for example, is quoted as saying that '[t]he conception is unbearable for me that, while the best young blood lose their lives at the front, the tainted asocial and unquestionably antisocial in the institutions have a guaranteed existence'. From R.E. Conot, *Justice at Nuremberg* (New York: Harper and Row Publishers, 1983), p. 206.

81 C.B. Davenport, 'Presidential address: The development of eugenics', in *A Decade of Progress in Eugenics: Scientific Papers of the Third International Congress of Eugenics* (Baltimore: Williams and Wilkins Company, 1934), p. 21.

82 'Autopsy puts boy in class of defectives', p. 1. For a more recent case that considers similar issues, see the Canadian case of Tracy Latimer, in D. Jenish, 'What would you do?' *Maclean's* 107:48 (1994), 16–24.

83 'Birth control is peril to race, says Osborn', p. 16.

84 Yukins, 'Feeble-minded white women', p. 164.

85 Kline, *Building a Better Race*, p. 16. Also see G. Bock, 'Racism and sexism in Nazi Germany: Motherhood, compulsory sterilization, and the state', *Signs* 8 (1983), 401–2.

86 See, for example, Robie, 'Selective sterilization for race culture', p. 207; Kline, *Building a Better Race*, pp. 148–50.

87 Roosevelt, 'Twisted eugenics', p. 311.

88 Kline, *Building a Better Race*, p. 8. Also see M.P. Daggett, 'Women: Building a better race', *World's Work* 25 (1912), 229–34.

89 This issue is additionally important because of the contemporary efforts by some groups in the United States to use Sanger to tie Planned Parenthood (the largest private provider of women's reproductive health services in the United States) to Nazism, using eugenics as a point of connection. This contention is inaccurate for a number of reasons, but primary because Sanger, though she shared some eugenic beliefs, was in no way a leading figure in the American eugenics movement.

90 Sanger, *The Pivot of Civilization*, chapter 4.

91 For the relationship between Sanger and eugenics, see E. Chesler, *Woman of Valor* (New York: Simon & Schuster, 1992), pp. 216–17, and E. Katz (ed.), *The Selected Papers of Margaret Sanger*, vol. I: *The Woman Rebel, 1900–1928* (Urbana: University of Illinois Press, 2003), pp. 252–5, 273–5, 313–5, 319–21.

92 Sanger believed that over-population, caused largely by unplanned pregnancies, was a major cause of war, as it induced nations to make efforts to expand their boundaries. See her *Women and the New Race* (New York: Blue Ribbon Books, 1920), chapter 13.

93 The eugenic perception of women as producers predated Hitler; see, for examples, M. Hillel and C. Henry, *Of Pure Blood*, trans. E. Mossbacher (New York: McGraw-Hill Book Co., 1976), p. 29, and Proctor, *Racial Hygiene*, p. 124.

94 Proctor, *Racial Hygiene*, p. 125.
95 Quoted in Weindling, *Health, Race and German Politics*, p. 445.
96 For example, see G.L. Mosse, *Nazi Culture: Intellectual, Cultural and Social Life in the Third Reich* (New York: Grosset & Dunlap, 1966), p. 46, and G. Sereny, *Into that Darkness: From Mercy Killing to Mass Murder* (London: Andre Deutsch, 1974), p. 55.
97 Hillel and Henry, *Of Pure Blood*, p. 165.
98 Baldwin, 'The psychology of mental deficiency', p. 92.
99 Ibid.
100 Weir noted that even up to the beginning of World War II 'there were "incubator baby sideshows", displaying premature and deformed infants for the curious public who paid to see the shows'. R.F. Weir, *Selective Nontreatment of Handicapped Newborns* (New York: Oxford University Press, 1984), p. 21. Also popular, and of even more recent vintage, were 'pickled punks', which were deformed fetuses that had been preserved in jars and displayed as a curiosity. See R. West, *Pickled Punks and Girlie Shows: A Life Spent on the Midways of America* (Atglen, PA: Schiffer Publishing, 2011).
101 Trent, *Inventing the Feeble Mind*, p. 157.
102 English, *Unnatural Selections*, p. 160.
103 Cole, 'The relation of philanthropy and medicine to race betterment', p. 499.
104 See S.L. Gilman, *Disease and Representation: Images of Illness from Madness to AIDS* (Ithaca: Cornell University Press, 1988).
105 A. Maxwell, *Picture Imperfect: Photography and Eugenics 1870–1940* (Brighton: Sussex Academic Press, 2008).
106 Ibid., p. 124.
107 Brave and Sylva, 'Exhibiting eugenics', p. 36.
108 Jackson, *The Borderland of Imbecility*, p. 92.
109 Ibid., p. 105.
110 Burleigh, *Death and Deliverance*, pp. 184, 196–7.
111 Pernick, *The Black Stork*, pp. 123–7.
112 Gould, *The Mismeasure of Man*, p. 171.
113 Whitney, *The Case for Sterilization*, p. 110.
114 D.S. Jordan, *The Heredity of Richard Roe* (Boston: American Unitarian Association, 1911), p. 81.
115 Robie, 'Selective sterilization for race culture', pp. 207–8.
116 It should be noted that when eugenicists and others talked about the increased tax burden caused by 'dependent' elements of the population, they were primarily discussing state and local taxes, as there were few federal 'welfare' policies in place at this time.
117 Whitney, 'A plea for the control of feeble-mindedness', p. 12.
118 J.H. Kempton, 'Sterilization for ten million Americans' (book review), *Journal of Heredity* 25 (1934), 418.
119 Sanger, *The Pivot of Civilization*, p. 100.

120   C.C. Little, 'President's address: Shall we live longer and should we?', in *Proceedings of the Third Race Betterment Conference* (Battle Creek, MI: Race Betterment Foundation, 1928), p. 13.

121   S.W. Evans, 'Eugenics on parade', *Eugenics* 3:10 (1930), 391.

122   Weindling, *Health, Race and German Politics*, pp. 442–5, 455.

123   Burleigh, *The Third Reich*, p. 391. Also see W. Frick, 'German population and race politics', trans. A. Hellmer, *Eugenical News* 19:2 (1934), 35; Lifton, *The Nazi Doctors*, p. 91.

124   Bock, 'Nazi sterilization and reproductive policies', p. 66; 'Case for sterilization', p. 136; Conot, *Justice at Nuremberg*, p. 205.

125   Weindling, *Health, Race and German Politics*, p. 545.

126   Friedlander, 'From "euthanasia" to the "final solution"', pp. 169–70.

127   W. McDougall, 'A national fund for a new plan of remuneration as a eugenic measure', in *Second International Congress of Eugenics*, vol. II (Baltimore: Williams & Wilkins Company, 1923), p. 62.

128   P. Popenoe, 'Should bachelors and fathers get the same pay?', *Eugenical News* 28:4 (1943), 52.

129   Stoddard, *The Revolt against Civilization*, p. 256.

130   Mencken, 'Utopia by sterilization', p. 408.

131   Ibid.

132   Ibid., 404. This proposal was strikingly similar to a more recent recommendation by the Nobel laureate William Shockley. See his 'Eugenic, or anti-dysgenic, thinking exercises'. Also see Ingle, *Who Should Have Children?*, pp. 96–7.

133   Whitney, *The Case for Sterilization*, pp. 275–6.

134   Deutsch, *Inventing America's 'Worst' Family*, p. 57.

135   Blatt, *Exodus from Pandomonium*, p. 18.

136   For example, see Burleigh's *Death and Deliverance* and Hillel and Henry's *Of Pure Blood*.

7

CONCLUSION[1]

> [E]ven while we loathe our meanness of spirit and narrow, bigoted views of what a human being can be, we are driven to starve ourselves of opportunities to enlarge variance in our lives. We shun those who are incompetent, infirm, palsied, different. We avoid those people as we try to avoid death itself; yet we know that to avoid them is to deny ourselves not only moral nourishment but the excitement and color that ultimately make life that much more worthwhile. Why do we do it?[2]

The forms of social control that were advanced by American advocates of eugenics (as well as, to a large degree, those in other nations) were more apt to be supported by the public and policymakers if the targets of control were portrayed as a growing threat to the rest of the population, and the dehumanizing metaphor themes that have been explicated in the previous chapters served as essential elements within the rhetorical arsenal of the eugenicists. These themes were employed to build a case for restricting human rights against a group that was seemingly non-threatening. Furthermore, as with many large-scale efforts to denigrate and control a devalued community subgroup, eugenicists had to strike a balance between adequately demarcating the prospective targets of eugenic control as a 'separate' class of humanity and at the same time augmenting the fear that such persons could pass as 'normal' and spread their degenerate characteristics throughout the population.

As a number of disability scholars (as well as those describing majority–minority relations in regard to other groups) have noted, various atypical traits or conditions present a dilemma for observers, who may be fascinated by the similarity between these 'different' persons and themselves while at the same time they are repulsed by the existential questions to which such divergence gives rise: questions, for example, regarding the nature of the 'human', the demarcation lines that relate to the provision of various rights, or, especially in the case of persons with disabilities, the temporal nature of our bodily integrity.[3]

There are several important implications of this research, and this final chapter will briefly delineate these. First, a crucial question about the eugenic period, or any alarm movement for that matter, relates to the nature of the various metaphor themes or sub-themes that are employed by those advocating control or restriction within the context of the movement. One might ask why specific stereotyped images come to be embraced, and whether contrasting metaphor images serve differing ends. These issues will be taken up in the first section of this chapter.

A second issue that relates to this first is the following: what was it about feeble-mindedness or moronity that caused it to become the central focal point of eugenic control? Certainly the preceding chapters have delineated this to some degree. Here, however, I try to set out and briefly analyze the major factors that served to focus special attention on persons who were diagnosed as feeble-minded. In contrast with the situation in many alarm movements (e.g., the various anti-communist movements in the United States), the search for a primary eugenic target could have led down multiple pathways. The newly developed moron classification, however, proved beneficial to the eugenic cause for a range of reasons.

Finally, the eugenic alarm era was not in any way unique in its negative view of persons with disabilities, and especially of those with mental, cognitive, or intellectual disabilities. It should be cautioned that one of the concerns about focusing on the pejorative aspects of eugenics is that this may play into one of the most dangerous misconceptions we may hold. This is the belief that the societal perception and treatment of persons with developmental disabilities (as well as, to varying degrees, persons with other types of disabilities) follows a relatively linear course throughout history. The view that is often embraced is that past treatment was largely horrendous, and that things have gradually but progressively improved within our more modern and humane culture and will likely continue on this path in the future. Even a cursory reading of history, however, would demonstrate that the treatment of persons with intellectual and mental disabilities has followed a largely vacillating course. I contend that the march of time has not been the primary ally of vulnerable groups, including those with developmental disabilities. More important have been such issues as relative economic, social, and political stability and the power and cohesion of consumer and advocacy groups. Rights (including the right to be regarded with a degree of respect) are rarely given to stigmatized groups outright; they are earned through self-advocacy. When they are given outright, this is almost always in a form of charity or altruism wherein a hierarchical ordering is maintained by such gratuitous measures.

These issues obviously pertain to, among other things, questions about the contemporary relevance of the eugenic alarm movement and what we have learned or should learn from this historical example, as well as the relationship of contemporary advancements in bioethics to past eugenic practices, and whether these should give us pause, as some have contended, to question whether a new era of eugenic control may assert itself and what form this may take.

Analysis of metaphor usage

In considering the nature of metaphor use for the purpose of dehumanization and the development of aversive formal or informal social policies, a few themes that were introduced in the previous chapters will be revisited and discussed in greater depth here. This section is primarily dedicated to the consideration of important issues that supported the utilization of specific metaphor themes within eugenic writing. In deconstructing the use of rhetoric within any alarm period, a key question obviously is: why were these particular themes or sub-themes chosen? A large variety of factors (cultural elements, prevailing societal fears, nature of or presumptions about source or target domains, background and bias of speakers or writers, access to publications or media outlets, forms of control desired, etc.) intersect to provide a potentially receptive environment for certain images. This complexity is heightened because dehumanizing rhetoric and images interconnect with one another across alarm periods. Elements of an image that were effectively utilized in a previous alarm period may be recycled for future use, redesigned to fit a somewhat different community subgroup.

There are a number of issues that come to the fore when we consider why certain metaphor themes came to be employed within the eugenic movement. First, the general academic or occupational orientation of supporters of eugenics obviously had much influence on the utilization of various themes. For example, the organism metaphor, with its focus on bodily integrity and 'pollution' from the outside, obviously struck a chord with many eugenicists who had a medical or biological background. Since institutions for persons with feeble-mindedness were largely administered by physicians, this obviously would include them. Animal metaphors certainly made sense to those eugenicists who had a zoological or animal biology background, and these included important leading figures in the movement such as Davenport, Laughlin, Michael Guyer, and Madison Grant. Additionally, many supporters, such as

Alexander Graham Bell, and Heinrich Himmler in Germany, came to their interest in eugenics partly through their own experiences in animal breeding.

As mentioned above, expanding interest in intelligence testing during the first decades of the century fostered the objectification of persons with intellectual disabilities as morons and, to use Gould's term, reified a 'condition' that many people assumed existed, but in a form that prior to the eugenic era they could not quite pin down. It supported the presumption that people could be given a seemingly objective, scientific procedure the results of which represented their inherent or 'native' intelligence.[4] It was important for eugenicists, especially those who were involved in testing and diagnosing subjects as morons or in the implementation of social control measures, to demonstrate that the decisions they carried were not based on subjective class or ethnic judgments but rather had an objective basis.

The eugenic era prospered during a period of intense professional and public interest in medical research, public health, prevention activities, and related domains. Concepts that pertained to the organism metaphor were in vogue during this period, and provided a modern way of framing eugenic goals that was in line with the general tenets of Progressivism. As noted previously, this was also an age where self-improvement and individual self-determination, especially in sexual matters, were highlighted. Eugenic proposals neatly connected with the increased responsibility that was placed on individuals (especially women) to understand and control their personal sexual development.[5] During the first decades of the twentieth century the undesired consequences of sexual behavior were matters that were coming increasingly under individual control. The mothers of unwanted children were no longer victims of happenstance, but rather agents of their own poor judgment.

Additionally, as was explained in Chapter 4, a central feature of feeblemindedness that predicated the employment of certain themes was the passive nature of such individuals. Unlike the images of anarchists, Jews, African-Americans, or Japanese immigrants that were predominant during the era of the eugenics movement, which generally presented them as engaging in a planned, or at least forcible, conspiratorial take-over of areas of trade or important geographic regions, those labeled as feeble-minded were depicted as unwittingly threatening the nation. They neither planned nor were even aware of the widespread harm they were perpetrating. While various aspects of the war metaphor were employed within the context of eugenic writing, these were (with a few exceptions) not overtly violent metaphoric images. The sexual behavior of the moron was not like the rapacious sexuality that is often attributed to the target group (e.g., African-American males in the United States, or Jews in Nazi Germany), but was just as destructive.

Why target feeble-mindedness?

In the context of the American eugenic era, the connection between worthless-ness, parasitism, and related themes seemed to be much more apparent in regard to persons with cognitive (or mental or emotional) disabilities than in those with physical ones. This is certainly not to imply that persons with physical dis-abilities were in any meaningful way embraced by the public during the period, or that there were not cultural elements that stigmatized and set apart such persons (e.g., 'freak shows'). However, those who supported eugenic control almost exclusively highlighted persons with feeble-mindedness as the principal target for control measures.[6] When they did discuss other disability groups, these primarily consisted of persons with various forms of mental illness.[7]

Additionally, though other target populations were included as potential subjects of control, these were normally vaguely defined groups (e.g., persons who were poor, lower-class or unemployed, the 'criminalistic' or 'hyper-sexual') whose problems were said to arise in large part from low mentality. Especially early in the eugenics movement, unfitness was described by a plethora of inexact and overlapping 'diagnoses', many of which were exceed-ingly vague. As Wright noted prior to the turn of the century,

> To a considerable extent these ... defective classes link into one another. It is hard to say whether a tramp is a pauper or a criminal ... A very large per cent of criminals become insane in prison or afterward. A considerable number of paupers become insane. The children of one class pass easily into the other class ... Here and there in our country, and in every other one, are knots of defectives all tangled up together, families closely related furnishing a whole population of criminals, idiots, and lunatics among themselves ... The interchangability of these defects is very clearly shown in these cases.[8]

Many early supporters of eugenic control simply spoke of defectives, unfit persons, or degenerates, and imprecise classifications such as moral insanity, moral imbecility, or moral defectiveness were developed in an effort to move in the direction of 'target clarity'. Most eugenicists felt that the various 'nega-tive' social behaviors largely were found in the same group of persons, and thus that focusing on one trait (e.g., alcoholism, prostitution, poverty) was not necessary. As noted previously, some writers simply talked of the bottom 10 percent of the population, a group that was characterized by a prepon-derance of interconnected negative traits. Henry Goddard noted that when Dugdale described the Juke family in the 1870s, its members experienced the full range of anti-social traits, with no clear pattern in regard to either a master dysgenic characteristic or even the certain transmission of hereditary traits.[9] Grandparents with epilepsy and insanity might have children who were identified as prostitutes and paupers, who themselves might sire children with feeble-mindedness and alcoholism.[10]

As the first decade of the twentieth century drew to a close, however, persons labeled as feeble-minded began to take center stage as the presumptive primary source of dysgenic evil within society, and eugenic unfitness came to be inextricably connected to moronity. The main reasons for this transformation included (a) the rediscovery of Mendel's laws, (b) the development of the intelligence test, (c) the involvement within the eugenics movement of institutional administrators, and, perhaps most importantly, (d) the flexibility of the 'moron' designation.

If, as many argued during the Progressive Era, environmental modifications could improve the status of 'unfit' individuals, then positive evolutionary growth could be fostered through the development of such modifications, referred to previously as 'euthenics'. Educational and environmental uplift, however, would do little to increase the capacity of such individuals and families if their 'impairments' were viewed as intrinsic and largely unalterable. For a society that, at least on its face, embraced fair play and human rights, the process of hereditary transmission was an important precursor for accepting an inherently pessimistic and non-egalitarian movement such as eugenics. The assumption that eugenic measures could greatly minimize feeble-mindedness was heightened by the unit-trait theory, to which many American eugenicists, especially early in the movement, held. This theory maintained that there was a one-to-one relationship between particular traits and genetic components.[11] Therefore, it was maintained, altering these traits through selective mating would be a feasible eugenic goal.

The intelligence test was developed in France at turn of the century by Alfred Binet, but came to be primarily employed in the United States at the beginning of the eugenics movement by psychologists such as Henry Goddard.[12] As noted previously, the test was crucial to the eugenic era in that it allowed for the supposedly scientific demarcation of the feeble-minded population, and especially the higher-functioning 'moron' subgroup. As Jessie Taft, a leading social worker of the time, wrote in 1918, '[t]here is no question that the swift rise of the mental test as a center of interest and experiment in applied psychology has had much to do with the growth of popular recognition of feeblemindedness as a social problem'.[13] Within a very short span of time, then, the convergence of hereditarianism and intelligence testing paved the way for the 'menace' of the feeble-minded. Moreover, this convergence came about at the same time as early eugenicists in the country such as Charles Davenport were attempting to focus attention on the need for eugenic planning. The image of the rapidly procreating destitute moron gave these eugenicists an image that they could employ as the focal point of the movement.

A bureaucratic infrastructure composed of a new brand of professionals (psychologists, psychiatrists, social workers, public health workers) and encompassing a broad range of social welfare and social control institutions had evolved around the turn of the century, pushed in large measure by urbanization. Many of those who ran, or held administrative positions within, institutions for persons with feeble-mindedness were important early leaders of the eugenics movement, and supported its focus on the 'moron'. Even before the rediscovery of Mendel's laws, some of them were already highlighting the importance of genetic transmission in the spread of moronity through the community. Martin Barr, for example, wrote in 1898 that '[n]o other class of defectives transmit ill with such certainty as the feeble-minded',[14] and Ernest Bicknell stated around the same time that '[t]he curse of feeble-mindedness descends from parents to child as no other defect does'.[15]

Certainly there were a variety of rationales (most of them well-meaning) for institutional administrators to support eugenic policies. Ironically, as noted in Chapter 3, a pessimistic view of moronity had taken hold during the Progressive Era, fostered in part by the fact that there was almost universal agreement among leaders in the field that earlier efforts to improve the mental capacity of such persons had failed, thus proving that such persons could not be brought within the 'mainstream' of the community.[16] While many institutionally based eugenicists certainly believed the fear they spread, many others no doubt saw intelligence testing, institutional-building, sterilization, and other forms of control as a way of expanding their authority and demonstrating the need for their professional expertise.

While supporters of eugenics often advocated for the control of other disability groups, none fitted their needs as well as those who were diagnosed as feeble-minded. The various forms of mental illness were not clearly understood at the time. Additionally, it was questioned even by many eugenicists whether mental illness was hereditary in nature. Freudian psychotherapy, which came to be embraced by many American psychiatrists and physicians during the eugenic era, held that mental health problems largely resulted from one's early upbringing, and thus did not principally have a genetic etiology. Moreover, these conditions came with no specific diagnostic tool, such as the intelligence test. Finally, many persons were not diagnosed as mentally ill until later in life, often after they already had borne children, and those with the most serious forms of insanity were, unlike persons believed to be feeble-minded, already institutionalized by the beginning of the eugenic era.[17]

The hereditary nature of other conditions, such as blindness and deafness, was also not well understood, and during the eugenic era individuals with sensory disorders were, for the most part, evaluated less pessimistically than in previous decades, largely because of the admiration for persons such as Helen Keller and Louis Braille. This is not to say, certainly, that they were treated in a humane manner, but only that they were not central targets for eugenic control in the United States. In her support for the infanticide of the Bollinger baby, Helen Keller highlighted the important distinction between persons diagnosed as morons and those with sensory or physical disabilities.[18] As noted in Chapter 3, the assumption that formed the philosophical foundation for much of eugenic thinking, and was important in the employment of various metaphor themes, was that the particular characteristic which principally defined the species Homo sapiens and set us apart from non-human animals was our mind, and that the humanity of those with diminished minds could be rightly called into question.[19]

As a number of eugenics scholars have noted, moronity provided the eugenicists with the best of both worlds. Basing the designation on a 'scientific' diagnostic tool allowed them to argue that they were not conditioning eugenic control on arbitrary personal or class judgments. This tool, however, was new (and thus malleable) enough to be manipulated in various ways. Additionally, persons diagnosed as feeble-minded generally had little formal education, and (especially in an era before informed consent guidelines) thus proved to be an easy target, as they were unlikely to attempt to self-advocate in an atmosphere where they were surrounded by physicians, psychologists, administrators, and other authority figures. The Carrie Buck case was symptomatic of the era, as Carrie's lawyer was actually chosen by and associated with the institution that wanted to have her sterilized.[20]

How moronity came to be socially constructed during the first few decades of the twentieth century is extraordinarily important in that this was a term that, when put forward by Goddard in 1910, was unknown and thus a 'linguistic vehicle' that could be shaped at will by eugenicists who wanted it to cover a broad range of undesirables.[21] Similarly, in Great Britain the term 'feeble-minded' (the British did not employ the term 'moron') 'possessed an "elastic capacity for embracing a whole array of existing social problems"'.[22]

The eugenic era and the 'new' eugenics: past as prologue?

The late Burton Blatt, one of the most respected advocates of persons with cognitive disabilities in the United States during the 1970s and 1980s, wrote in 1987 that he was 'troubled that there lingers yet deep and widespread feelings that it [the eugenics movement] wasn't so much a case of giving up the dream as missing the opportunity'. 'I am troubled', Blatt wrote, 'that the philosophy, if not the practice, of human eugenics has strong representation in our culture'.[23] Blatt was in no way alone in stating this fear. Hugh Gregory Gallagher, in an article on hate crimes against persons with disabilities entitled 'Slapping up spastics', contended, '[i]t is my conviction that the underlying assumption that made possible the killing of upwards of two hundred thousand disabled German citizens in the 1930s and 1940s are still widely held, not just in Germany but throughout the Western industrialized world'.[24] He continued, 'it is my conclusion the underlying psychological attitudes and assumptions concerning the worth and place of disabled people in society have not changed very much over fifty years'.[25]

These quotations are representative of a number of authors who have expressed similar fears, especially within the disability community. These concerns lead us to one of the more intriguing and fundamentally important questions that is often posed in relation to the eugenic era (or any alarm period, for that matter). This is the consideration of the possibility that repressive episodes of the past may be revisited in the future in some guise. We may question what specific events, known or unknown fears, social or economic incentives, and other factors precipitated the original period, the degree to which a somewhat similar confluence of events may occur, and in what ways the period might bear a resemblance to what preceded it.

Hasian, in his book *The Rhetoric of Eugenics in Anglo-American Thought*, discussed the contemporary relevance of the eugenic period. He noted that:

> The celebration story treats eugenics as a pernicious doctrine invoked by the misguided, while the lamentation tale treats every scientist or practitioner interested in germ theory as a villain who is duping the public. Both of these orientations run into difficulties when we consider the possibility that a substantial percentage of the Anglo-American public believed (and still believe) in the tenets of eugenics.[26]

In Hasian's 'celebration story', supporters of eugenics were (largely) well-meaning but misguided individuals who really believed that they could solve the world's problems by controlling procreation. Such a story, one might contend, carries with it the belief that eugenics and controlled human breeding could not be revisited because we now know much more about the nature of genetics than was known at the time, and we therefore understand the foolishness of attempting to guide our evolutionary path. Hasian's 'lamentation tale' focuses on the notion that American eugenicists were all pseudo-Nazis who were taken much too seriously and allowed to have more control than they should have had. Accepting this view requires a rather limited degree of understanding of the eugenic era and those who supported it.[27] The fallacious belief that devolves from either of these two views is that we now live in a more enlightened era that would refuse to fall for such rubbish.

According to both Garland Allen and Elof Carlson, the temptation to find rationalizations to restrict the rights or even the lives of persons with disabilities rises and falls in part on the basis of such issues as the economy and other large-scale challenges (e.g. natural or man-made disasters, war) that a nation may be facing. Carlson wrote that:

> During the emotional climate of a tense period in a nation's history, the normal restraints that protect political, religious, or racial opponents as fundamentally people like us can be shattered, and the justification to destroy a hated or dangerous population can be overwhelming. Atrocities against civilians, like wars themselves, after many years have elapsed, may seem historically archaic and in times of peace, good will, and prosperity, an impossibility. A changing troubled economy, new social upheavals, and international conflict can suddenly trigger inappropriate hostility leading to the deaths of innocent groups.[28]

Allen for his part contends that the United States is already beginning to 're-walk those paths of trying to solve our social problems with scientific panaceas'. 'A new eugenics movement would', he continues, 'be called by a different name, but an era of similar economic and social conditions and a similar political response – our current philosophy of "cost-effectiveness" or "the bottom line" – has already arrived'.[29] It should be noted that Allen's comments were written at a time when the economic conditions within the United States were, to put it mildly, quite good compared with those of recent years. In order to assess the potential for a 'new eugenic' era in the United States, it makes sense to turn our attention to the area where this controversy primarily rages: the application of and ethical issues pertaining to new genetic technology, and the potential impact that this may have on our perception and treatment of persons with disabilities.

The recent expansion and practical application of genetic research has fostered, depending on one's perception, utopian dreams of a world without disability or dystopian nightmares of a world that is both largely devoid and highly contemptuous of persons with disabilities. Genetic counseling, new methods of reproduction, the pre-implantation screening of embryos, implementation of technology based on the Human Genome Project, and other recent (and potentially future) genetic practices are at times cited (almost always by opponents or those seeking controls on such methods) as a form of 'new eugenics'. Some disability rights groups and advocates have even compared genetic innovations, especially genetic testing coupled with abortion, to a form of cultural or minority-group genocide.[30]

Whether certain reproductive technologies and breeding practices can rightly be considered eugenic is often questioned on several grounds. Most importantly, whereas previous practices such as sterilization and restrictive marriage were state-sponsored, contemporary decisions are driven largely by prospective parents themselves. Such practices are widely viewed as an important element of parental self-determination. Supporters argue that non-directive counseling provides potential parents with a realistic awareness of the child's limitations and the possible impact on the family, and leaves the decision in their hands. One could, in fact, argue that governmental restrictions of such research or its application would be ideologically reminiscent of those earlier forms of eugenics where the breeding opportunities of persons were controlled by the state.

Another important issue here is that the decisions that are made by parents are largely contingent upon their assumption of the issues that may arise in relation to the child's presence within the family. This includes the perceived impact on the parents' social or occupational opportunities or on siblings, the child's presumptive quality of life, financial considerations, and so on. One would assume that more broad societal issues, such as the need to protect the larger gene pool or support the positive evolution of the species, seldom arise in the course of such decision-making. While eugenics, therefore, was a program designed to have large-scale impact on a population, it would appear that this is not the case with contemporary family-based decisions. It is certainly possible, however, that governmental support for and access to genetic testing and certain related medical procedures could be motivated in part by such demographic or macroeconomic considerations.

Importantly, some of the contentions noted above have been questioned by certain disability advocacy groups and other opponents of widespread testing and application of genetic procedures. Even if parental self-determination is viewed as the driving force behind the development and utilization of such technological advances, such decisions do not take place within a socio-cultural vacuum, but rather against the backdrop of and influenced by a society that is overly pessimistic and at times even resentful or fearful of persons with disabilities. Additionally, the powerful medical industry in the nation plays a highly influential role in framing disability for prospective parents, and also has a vested interest in the widespread development and deployment of relevant technology.

Adding complexity to these issues is the fact that 'disability' lends itself to a wide variety of conditions. Even the staunchest opponents of fetal selection would be hard pressed to disallow testing in the most extreme cases, as, for example, in the case of Tay–Sachs disease or anencephaly. On the other hand, opponents of large-scale testing might question why it is taken for granted as appropriate in cases of Down syndrome children, where little apparent pain or discomfort is involved and the person may live a fairly independent life. Further muddying the waters, even a specific disability has a wide range of effects on unique individuals, which relate not only to the differential physiological impacts of the condition, but to a host of additional psychological, social, life-stage, and environmental elements.[31] To some degree, moreover, decisions about whether to utilize existing technology and what to do with the information gained will relate to cultural assumptions that arise in part from media and metaphoric representations of individuals with disabilities.

One might argue that persons with disabilities receive two important 'meta-messages' about the nature of disability within American culture, and that these messages directly contradict one another. The first message is that these persons are accepted as full citizens within the community, that any form of discrimination or prejudice against them is to be resoundingly condemned by society at large, and that the community should do its part to accommodate individual needs. The second message is that fetuses who have the same disabilities as these persons are undesirable, or at least that the parental decision to prevent the birth of such a child is a perfectly reasonable one, not to be interfered with.[32] This latter message may carry with it an important meaning of how others within the community with such conditions are valued, and may diminish the veracity of the former message.

The contemporary influence of the eugenics movement in the United States, however, has continued in other spheres outside of bioethics. Just as involuntary sterilization[33] in North Carolina and other areas of the South was transformed over time from a program to control persons diagnosed as feeble-minded to one to control those receiving 'welfare' payments, discussions continue surrounding the overlap between various social policies (e.g., regarding taxation) and differential reproduction. The 1990s Norplant debate whereby recommendations were made to provide financial incentives for women on public assistance who were implanted with the long-lasting birth control is typical of this.[34] As Patrick Ryan noted, eugenics was and continues to be 'a constituent part of an ongoing American poverty discourse'.[35] As was the case a century ago, eugenic programs may evolve almost imperceptibly to target an increasing range of devalued community groups.

Regardless of where one stands on these complex ethical and moral issues, the continued vulnerability of persons with intellectual and other disabilities cannot easily be disputed. It is my hope that this study and others like it will at least give us pause when we consider the treatment of marginalized groups, and challenge us to question the basis on which important policy decisions restricting their rights are made. We live in a social and political climate that seems increasingly to embrace style over substance, and mythology, stereotypes, often meaningless rhetoric, and talking points over the ability to engage honestly in critical thought about complex issues. This is a problematic trend in any case, but is especially troubling when human rights are at stake.

While we would like to believe that rhetoric like that detailed in this book is largely a thing of the past, most readers have probably been struck by the similarities between some of the themes described here and the means by which various groups are frequently framed today. Additionally, advancements in computer and other forms of communication technology have left us swamped by 'information overload'. As we find it increasingly difficult to process, evaluate, and organize the extensive amount of information presented to us, we will continue to look for shortcuts: ways to 'understand' the world that take as little time and effort as possible. In other words, there will likely be an expanding use of metaphors and similar forms of rhetorical understanding in conjunction with these current and future technological advancements. It is vitally important, therefore, that those who advocate fair treatment of vulnerable populations find effective ways of deconstructing damaging metaphors, shed light on the historic precursors that undergird their use and support their potential effectiveness, and widely disseminate this knowledge in an effort to counterbalance dehumanizing or threatening images.

Notes

1 Sections of this chapter were originally published in the author's 'Eugenics, genetics and the minority group model of disabilities'.

2 Blatt, *The Conquest of Mental Retardation*, p. 329.

3 See Shakespeare, 'Cultural representation of disabled people'; Fiedler, *Freaks*; R.G. Thomson, 'Seeing the disabled: Visual rhetorics of disability in popular photography', in P.K. Longmore and L. Umansky (eds.), *The New Disability History* (New York: New York University Press, 2001), pp. 335–74.

4 In chapter 5 of *The Mismeasure of Man*, Gould describes how cultural information was used to measure supposedly inherent intelligence.

5 Certainly there was widespread disagreement within society about such 'sexual empowerment'. Before the Progressive Era, however, even public debates about such topics were frowned upon or viewed as a form of obscenity.

6 This is in contrast to Nazi Germany, where insanity was highlighted alongside moronity as a primary target of eugenic control. Nazi propaganda drew little distinction between the two.

7 O'Brien and Bundy, 'Reaching beyond the moron.'

8   Wright, 'The defective classes', p. 227.
9   Goddard, *The Kallikak Family*. Of course, one of the reasons why Dugdale did not focus on hereditary transmission is that his study preceded the rediscovery of Mendel's laws.
10 One theory related to this belief was that of degeneration, which was held by a number of early eugenicists. Degeneration theory held that dysgenic persons (especially those who mated with other such individuals) bore children who were somewhat more 'defective' than themselves, and that this trend continued for multiple generations, ending with progeny having profound mental retardation.
11 See, for example, Smith, *Minds Made Feeble*, pp. 64–5.
12 Gould, *The Mismeasure of Man*, chapter 5.
13 Taft, 'Supervision of the feebleminded in the community', pp. 543–4.
14 Barr, 'Defective children', p. 483.
15 Bicknell, 'Custodial care of the adult feeble-minded', p. 81.
16 Trent, *Inventing the Feeble Mind*.
17 It should be noted, however, that even though persons with mental illness were not primary subjects of eugenic rhetoric in the United States, such persons were greatly impacted by eugenic policies, especially involuntary sterilization. A substantial percentage of the victims of eugenic sterilization laws were individuals thought to have various forms of mental illness. See O'Brien and Bundy, 'Reaching beyond the moron'.
18 As discussed in Chapter 3, Keller noted that the decision was in keeping with the need to '[weed] the human garden'. See Keller, 'Physicians' juries for defective babies'.
19 See O'Brien, 'Speciesism revisited', or Shakespeare, 'Cultural representation for disabled people'.
20 Smith and Nelson, *The Sterilization of Carrie Buck*.
21 In a 1910 article Goddard wrote: 'the other word proposed [for those children who were not "normal" but also did not quality as imbeciles] is a Greek word meaning foolish, "moronia", and these children might be called "morons"'. He continued, 'fool or foolish in the English sense exactly describes this group of children ... We should have moron for the noun, moronia for the condition, moronic for the adjective, and so it would seem to answer every requirement'. See 'Four hundred feeble-minded children classified by the Binet method', *Journal of Psycho-Asthenics* 15 (1910), 27.
22 Quoted in Jackson, *The Borderland of Imbecility*, p. 149.
23 Blatt, *The Conquest of Mental Retardation*, p. 320.
24 H.G. Gallagher, '"Slapping up spastics": The persistence of social attitudes toward people with disabilities', *Issues in Law & Medicine* 10 (1995), 401.
25 Ibid., p. 414.
26 Haskin, *The Rhetoric of Eugenics*, p. 5.
27 Also see C.S. Burke and C.J. Castaneda, 'The public and private history of eugenics: An introduction', *Public Historian* 29: 3 (2007), 8.

28 Carlson, *The Unfit*, p. 353.
29 G.E. Allen, 'Science misapplied: The eugenic age revisited', *Technology Review* 99:6 (1996), 29.
30 See, for example, M. Saxton, 'Why members of the disability community oppose prenatal diagnosis and selective abortion', in E. Parens and A. Asch (eds.), *Prenatal Testing and Disability Rights* (Washington, DC: Georgetown University Press, 2000), 147–64.
31 R.P Marinelli and A.E. Dell Orto (eds.), *The Psychological and Social Impact of Disability*, 3rd edn. (New York: Springer Publishing Company, 1991); Parens and Asch (eds.), *Prenatal Testing and Disability Rights*.
32 While some may argue, again, that these are personal decisions of the prospective parents, it should be noted that as a community we might be wary of allowing such decisions when they are based on gender (e.g., the aborting of female fetuses) or another 'suspect category' (e.g., if in the future a genetic link to homosexuality was found, and this could be determined through prenatal testing, would it be appropriate to 'select' for this quality?).
33 As should be clear from some of the preceding discussion, it is very difficult to adequately determine where the division between 'voluntary' and 'involuntary' sterilization lies. If, for example, as person is not forced to become sterilized but chooses to do so in order to gain a financial incentive, is the decision truly voluntary?
34 For more on Norplant and incentives, see A. Cockburn, 'Social cleansing', *New Statesman and Society* (August 1994), 16–18, and M. Henley, 'The creation and perpetuation of the mother/body myth: Judicial and legislative enlistment of Norplant', *Buffalo Law Review* 41 (1993), 734–59.
35 Ryan, 'Six blacks from home', p. 274.

Bibliography

Books and book chapters

Aly, G., Chroust, P. and Pross, C. *Cleansing the Fatherland: Nazi Medicine and Racial Hygiene*, trans. B. Cooper. Baltimore: Johns Hopkins University Press, 1994.

Baker, L.H. *Race Improvement or Eugenics: A Little Book on a Great Subject*. New York: Dodd, Mead and Company, 1912.

Beecher, H.K. *Research and the Individual*. Boston: Little, Brown and Co, 1970.

Biddiss, M.D. *Father of Racist Ideology: The Social and Political Thought of Count Gobineau*. London: Weidenfeld and Nicolson, 1970.

Black, E. *War against the Weak: Eugenics and America's Campaign to Create a Master Race*. New York: Four Walls Eight Windows, 2003.

Blatt, B. *Exodus from Pandomonium*. Boston: Allyn and Bacon, Inc., 1970.

——. *The Conquest of Mental Retardation*. Austin, TX: Pro-Ed, 1987.

Boas, F. 'Instability of human types', in G.W. Stocking, Jr. (ed.), *The Shaping of American Anthropology 1883–1911: A Franz Boas Reader*. New York: Basic Books, Inc., 1974, pp. 214–8.

Bock, G. 'Nazi sterilization and reproductive policies', in *Deadly Medicine: Creating the Master Race*. Washington, DC: United States Holocaust Memorial Museum, 2004, pp. 61–88.

Bowler, P.J. *Evolution: The History of an Idea*. Berkeley, CA: University of California Press, 1984.

Breitman, R. *The Architect of Genocide: Himmler and the Final Solution*. New York: Alfred A. Knopf, 1991.

Brennan, W. *Dehumanizing the Vulnerable: When Word Games Take Lives*. Chicago: Loyola University Press, 1995.

Brigham, C.C. *A Study of American Intelligence*. London: Princeton University Press, 1923.

Bruce, R.V. *Bell: Alexander Graham Bell and the Conquest of Solitude*. Boston: Little, Brown and Co., 1973.

Burbank, L. *The Training of the Human Plant*. New York: Century Co., 1907.

Burleigh, M. *Death and Deliverance: 'Euthanasia' in Germany 1900–1945*. Cambridge: Cambridge University Press, 1994.

——. *The Third Reich: A New History*. New York: Hill and Wang, 2000.

Calavita, K. *U.S. Immigration Law and the Control of Labor: 1820–1924*. London: Academic Press, Inc., 1984.

Carden, M.L. *Oneida: Utopian Community to Modern Corporation*. Baltimore: Johns Hopkins University Press, 1969.

Carlson, E.A. *The Unfit: A History of a Bad Idea*. Cold Spring Harbor, NY: Cold Spring Harbor Laboratory Press, 2001.

Chamberlain, H.S. *Foundations of the Nineteenth Century*, trans. J. Lees. New York: John Lane Co., 1913.

Chase, A. *The Legacy of Malthus*. New York: Alfred A. Knopf, 1977.

Chatterton-Hill, G. *Heredity and Selection in Sociology*. London: Adam and Charles Black, 1907.

Chesler, E. *Woman of Valor*. New York: Simon & Schuster, 1992.

Childs, D.J. *Modernism and Eugenics: Woolf, Eliot, Yeats, and the Culture of Degeneration*. Cambridge: Cambridge University Press, 2001.

Chorover, S. *From Genesis to Genocide*. Cambridge, MA: M.I.T. Press, 1979.

Cogdell, C. *Eugenic Design: Streamlining America in the 1930s*. Philadelphia: University of Pennsylvania Press, 2004.

Cohn, N. *Warrant for Genocide: The Myth of the Jewish World-Conspiracy and the Protocols of the Elders of Zion*. New York: Harper & Row Publishers, 1966.

Conot, R.E. *Justice at Nuremberg*. New York: Harper and Row Publishers, 1983.

Cuddy, L.A. and Roche, C.M. (eds.). *Evolution and Eugenics in American Literature and Culture, 1880-1940*. Lewisburg: Bucknell University Press, 2003.

Curran, T.J. *Xenophobia and Immigration, 1820-1930*. Boston: Twayne Publishers, 1975.

Currell, S. and Cogdell C. (eds.). *Popular Eugenics: National Efficiency and American Mass Culture in the 1930s*. Athens: Ohio University Press, 2006.

Davenport, C.B. *Heredity in Relation to Eugenics*. New York: Henry Holt and Company, 1911.

——. 'The eugenics programme and progress in its achievement', in *Eugenics: Twelve University Lectures*. New York: Dodd, Mead and Company, 1914, pp. 1–14.

Davies, S.P. *Social Control of the Mentally Deficient*. New York: Thomas Y. Crowell Company Publishers, 1930.

Degler, C.N. *In Search of Human Nature*. New York: Oxford University Press, 1991.

De Gobineau, A. *The Inequality of Human Races*, trans. A. Collins, reprint edn. Los Angeles: Noontide Press, 1966.

Deutsch, A. *The Mentally Ill in America: A History of their Care and Treatment from Colonial Times*. Garden City, NY: Doubleday, Doran and Co., 1938.

——. *The Shame of the States*, reprint edn. New York: Arno Press, 1973.

Deutsch, N. *Inventing America's 'Worst' Family: Eugenics, Islam, and the Fall and Rise of the Tribe of Ishmael*. Berkelely, CA: University of California Press, 2009.

De Vos, G.A. and Suárez-Orozco, M.M. 'Sacrifice and the experience of power', in G.A. De Vos and M.M. Suárez-Orozco (eds.), *Status Inequality: The Self in Culture*. Newbury Park, CA: Sage Publications, 1990, pp. 120–47.

Dix, D. 'Memorial to the legislature of Massachusetts, 1843', in M. Rosen, G.R. Clark, and M.S. Kivitz (eds.), *The History of Mental Retardation: Collected Papers*, vol. I. Baltimore: University Park Press, 1976, pp. 4–30.

Dombrowski, D.A. *Babies and Beasts: The Argument from Marginal Cases*. Urbana: University of Illinois Press, 1997.

Douglas, M. *Purity and Danger: An Analysis of the Concepts of Pollution and Taboo*. London: Routledge and Kegan Paul, 1966.

duBois, P. *Centaurs and Amazons: Women and the Pre-History of the Great Chain of Being*. Ann Arbor: University of Michigan Press, 1991.

DuBois, P.H. *A History of Psychological Testing*. Boston: Allyn and Bacon, Inc., 1970.

Dugdale, R.L. *The Jukes: A Study in Crime, Pauperism, Disease, and Heredity*, 4th edn. New York: G.P. Putnam's Sons, 1910.

East, E.M. *Heredity and Human Affairs*. New York: Charles Scribner's Sons, 1927.

English, D.K. *Unnatural Selections: Eugenics in American Modernism and the Harlem Renaissance*. Chapel Hill: University of North Carolina Press, 2004.

Fairchild, H.P. *Immigration: A World Movement and its American Significance*. New York: Macmillan Company, 1926.

Fancher, R.E. *The Intelligence Men: Makers of the I.Q. Controversy*. New York: W.W. Norton and Co., 1985.

Fielder, L. *Freaks: Myths and Images of the Secret Self*, reprint edn. New York: Doubleday, 1993.

Fleming, G. *Hitler and the Final Solution*. Berkeley, CA: University of California Press, 1982.

Fletcher, J. *The Ethics of Genetic Control*. Garden City, NY: Anchor Books, 1974.

Forrest, D.W. *Francis Galton: The Life and Work of a Victorian Genius*. New York: Taplinger Publishing Co., Inc., 1974.

Foucault, M. *Madness and Civilization*, trans. R. Howard. New York: Vintage Books, 1965.

Freire, P. *Pedagogy of the Oppressed*, trans. M.B. Ramos, reprint edn. New York: Continuum, 1986.

Friedlander, H. 'From "euthanasia" to the "final solution"', in *Deadly Medicine: Creating the Master Race*. Washington DC: United States Holocaust Memorial Museum, 2004, pp. 155–84.

Fries K. (ed.). *Staring Back: The Disability Experience from the Inside Out*. New York: Penguin Putman, Inc., 1997.

Galton, F. *Hereditary Genius*. New York: D. Appleton and Co., 1870.

——. *Inquiries into Human Faculty and its Development*, New York: E.P. Dutton & Co., 1907.

——. *Essays in Eugenics*, reprint edn. Washington, DC: Scott Townsend Publishers, 1996.

——. 'Eugenics as a factor in religion', in Galton, *Essays in Eugenics*, pp. 68–70.

Gasman, D. *The Scientific Origins of National Socialism: Social Darwinism in Ersnt Haeckel and the German Monist League*. New York: American Elsevier Inc., 1971.

Gilman, S.L. *Disease and Representation: Images of Illness from Madness to AIDS*. Ithaca: Cornell University Press, 1988.

Goddard, H.H. *Feeble-Mindedness: Its Causes and Consequences*. New York: Macmillan Co., 1914.

——. *The Kallikak Family*. New York: Arno Press, 1912.

Goffman, E. *Asylums: Essays on the Social Situation of Mental Patients and Other Inmates*. Garden City, NY: Anchor Books, 1961.

——. *Stigma*. Englewood Cliffs, NJ: Prentice-Hall, Inc., 1963.

Goldhagen, D.J. *Hitler's Willing Executioners: Ordinary Germans and the Holocaust*. New York: Alfred A. Knopf, 1996.

Goodey, C.F. 'The psychopolitics of learning and disability in seventeenth-century thought', in D. Wright and A. Dingby (eds.), *From Idiocy to Mental Deficiency: Historical Perspectives on People with Learning Disabilities*. London: Routledge, 1996, pp. 93–117.

Gosney, E.S., and Popenoe, P. *Sterilization for Human Betterment*, reprint edn. New York: Macmillan Company, 1980.

Gould, S.J. *The Panda's Thumb*. New York: W.W. Norton and Co., 1980.

——. *Ever Since Darwin: Reflections of Natural History*. New York: W.W. Norton and Co., 1981.

——. *The Mismeasure of Man*. New York: W.W. Norton and Co., 1981.

——. *Dinosaur in a Haystack*. New York: Harmony Books, 1995.

Grant, M. *The Passing of the Great Race: Or, the Racial Basis of European History*. New York: Charles Scribner's Sons, 1916.

——. *The Conquest of a Continent*. New York: Charles Scribner's Sons, 1933.

Gulick, S.J. *The American Japanese Problem*. New York: Charles Scribner's Sons, 1914.

Guyer, M.F. *Being Well-Born: An Introduction to Heredity and Eugenics*. Indianapolis: Bobbs-Merrill Company, 1927.

Hadden, W.J. *The Science of Eugenics and Sex Life*, ed. C.H. Robinson 2nd edn. W.R. Vansant, 1914.

Hague, W.G. *The Eugenic Marriage*, vol. I. New York: Review of Reviews Company, 1914.

Haldane, J.B.S. *Heredity and Politics*. New York: W.W. Norton & Company, 1938.

Haller, M.H. *Eugenics: Hereditarian Attitudes in American Thought*. New Brunswick: Rutgers University Press, 1963.

Hasian, M.A., Jr. *The Rhetoric of Eugenics in Anglo-American Thought*. Athens, GA: University of Georgia Press, 1996.

Hertzler, J.O. *The History of Utopian Thought*. New York: Cooper Square Publishers, Inc., 1965.

Hilberg, R. *The Destruction of the European Jaws*, reprint edn. Chicago: Quadrangle Books, 1967.

Hillel, M. and Henry, C. *Of Pure Blood*, trans. E. Mossbacher. New York: McGraw-Hill Book Co., 1976.

Hitler, A. *Mein Kampf*, trans. R. Manheim, reprint edn. Boston: Houghton Mifflin Co., 1971.

Höhne, H. *The Order of the Death's Head*, trans. R. Barry. New York: Ballantine Books, 1969.

Holmes, S.J. *The Eugenic Predicament*. New York: Harcourt, Brace and Company, 1933.

——. *Human Genetics and its Social Importance*. New York: McGraw-Hill Book Co., Inc., 1936.

Hooton, E.A. *Apes, Men and Morons.* New York: G.P. Putnam's Sons, 1937.

——. *Crime and the Man,* reprint edn. New York: Greenwood Press, 1968.

——. *The American Criminal: An Anthropological Study,* reprint edn. New York: Greenwood Press, 1969.

Horsman, R. *Race and Manifest Destiny: The Origins of American Racial Anglo Saxonism.* Cambridge, MA: Harvard University Press, 1981.

Huntington, E. *Tomorrow's Children: The Goal of Eugenics.* New York: John Wiley & Sons, Inc., 1935.

Huntington, E. and Whitney, L.F., *The Builders of America.* New York: William Morrow and Co., 1927.

Ingle, D.J. *Who Should Have Children?* Indianapolis: Bobbs-Merrill Co., Inc., 1973.

The International Jew: The World's Foremost Problem, vol. IV. Dearborn, MI: Dearborn Independent, 1922.

Iseman, M.S. *Race Suicide.* New York: Cosmopolitan Press, 1912.

Jackson, M. *The Borderland of Imbecility: Medicine, Society and the Fabrication of the Feeble Mind in Late Victorian and Edwardian England.* Manchester: Manchester University Press, 2000.

Jefferis, B.G. and J.L. Nichols. *Safe Counsel or Practical Eugenics,* 37th edn. Naperville, IL: J.L. Nichols & Co., 1924.

Jennings, H.S. *The Biological Basis of Human Nature.* New York: W.W. Norton & Co., 1930.

Jordan, D.S. *The Heredity of Richard Roe.* Boston: American Unitarian Association, 1911.

The Kallikaks of Kansas: Report of the Kansas Commission on Provision for the Feebleminded. Topeka: Kansas State Printing Plant, 1919.

Kamin, L.J. *The Science and Politics of I.Q.* Potomac, MD: Lawrence Erlbaum Association, 1974.

Katz, E. (ed.). *The Selected Papers of Margaret Sanger,* vol. I: *The Woman Rebel, 1900–1928.* Urbana: University of Illinois Press, 2003.

Keen, S. *Faces of the Enemy: Reflections of the Hostile Imagination.* San Francisco: Harper and Row, 1986.

Kevles, D.J. *In the Name of Eugenics.* New York: Alfred A. Knopf., 1985.

Kintner, E.W. (ed.). *Trial of Alfons Klein, Adolf Wahlmann, Heinrich Ruoff, Karl Willig, Adolf Merkle, Irmgard Huber, and Philipp Blum (the Hadamar Trial).* London: William Hodge and Company, Limited, 1949.

Klaw, S. *Without Sin: The Life and Death of the Oneida Community.* New York: Penguin Press, 1993.

Klein, A.E. *Threads of Life: Genetics from Aristotle to D.N.A.,* Garden City, NJ: Natural History Press, 1970.

Kline, W. *Building a Better Race: Gender, Sexuality and Eugenics from the Turn of the Century to the Baby Boom.* Berkeley: University of California Press, 2001.

Kostir, M.S. *The Family of Sam Sixty.* Mansfield, OH: Press of Ohio State Reformatory, 1916.

Kraut, A.M. *Silent Travelers: Germs, Genes and the 'Immigrant Menace'*. New York: Basic Books, 1994.

Kuhl, S. *The Nazi Connection: Eugenics, American Racism, and German National Socialism*. New York: Oxford University Press, 1994.

Lakoff, G. *Moral Politics: What Conservatives Know that Liberals Don't*. Chicago and London: University of Chicago Press, 1996.

—— and Johnson, M. *Metaphors We Live By*, 2nd edn. Chicago: University of Chicago Press, 2003.

Lane, H. *The Wild Boy of Aveyron*, New York: Bantam Books, 1976.

Larson, E.J. *Sex, Race and Science: Eugenics in the Deep South*. Baltimore: Johns Hopkins University Press, 1996.

Laughlin, H.H. 'The control of trends in the racial composition of the American people', in M. Grant and C.S. Davison (eds.), *The Alien in Our Midst*. New York: Galton Publishing Co., Inc., 1930, pp. 158–79.

Le Chêne, E. *Mauthausen: The History of a Death Camp*. London: Methuen & Co. Ltd., 1971.

Leiser, E. *Nazi Cinema*, trans. G. Mander and D. Wilson. New York: Macmillan Publishing Co., Inc., 1974.

Lerner, M. (ed.). *The Mind and Faith of Justice Holmes*. Boston: Little, Brown and Company, 1943.

Levin, M.B. *Political Hysteria in America*. New York: Basic Books, Inc., 1971.

Lifton, R.J. *The Nazi Doctors: Medical Killing and the Psychology of Genocide*. New York: Basic Books, Inc., 1986.

Livneh, H. 'On the origins of negative attitudes toward people with disabilities', in R. Marinelli and A.D. Dell Orto (eds.), *The Psychological and Social Impact of Disability*, 3rd edn. New York: Springer Publishing Company, 1991, pp. 181–96.

Lombroso, C. *Crime: Its Causes and Remedies*, trans. H.P. Horton, Montclair, NJ: Patterson Smith, 1968.

Lovejoy, A.O. *The Great Chain of Being*. Cambridge, MA: Harvard University Press, 1966.

Lowenthal, L. and Guterman, N. *Prophets of Deceit: A Study of Techniques of the American Agitator*, 2nd edn. Palo Alto, CA: Pacific Books, 1970.

Ludmerer, K.M. *Genetics and American Society*. Baltimore: Johns Hopkins University Press, Baltimore, 1972.

Malthus, T.R. *An Essay on the Principle of Population*, vol. II, reprint edn. New York: Dutton, 1967.

Marinelli, R.P. & Dell Orto, A.E. (eds.). *The Psychological and Social Impact of Disability*, 3rd edn. New York: Springer Publishing Company, 1991.

Marrus, M.R. *The Unwanted*. Oxford: Oxford University Press, 1985.

Maxwell, A. *Picture Imperfect: Photography and Eugenics 1870–1940*. Brighton: Sussex Academic Press, 2008.

McKim, W.D. *Heredity and Human Progress*. New York: G.P. Putnam's Sons, 1901.

McPhee, J. *The Pine Barrens*, 2nd edn. New York: Farrar, Straus, & Giroux, 1968.

Miller, M.D. *Terminating the 'Socially Inadequate': The American Eugenicists and the*

German Race Hygienists, California to Cold Spring Harbor, Long Island to Germany. Commack, NY: Malamud-Rose, Publisher, 1996.

Miller, W.I. *The Anatomy of Disgust.* Cambridge, MA: Harvard University Press, 1997.

Mosse, G.L. *Nazi Culture: Intellectual, Cultural and Social Life in the Third Reich.* New York: Grosset & Dunlap, 1966.

Müller-Hill, B. *Murderous Science: Elimination by Scientific Selection of Jews, Gypsies and Others: Germany 1933–1945,* trans. G.R. Fraser. New York: Oxford University Press, 1988.

Musolff, A. *Metaphor and Political Discourse: Analogical Reasoning in Debates about Europe.* Palgrave Press, 2004.

Nelkin, D. and Tancredi, L. *Dangerous Diagnostics: The Social Power of Biological Information.* New York: Basic Books, 1989.

Newbeck, P. *Virginia hasn't Always been for Lovers: Interracial Marriage Bans and the Case of Richard and Mildred Loving.* Carbondale, IL: Southern Illinois University Press, 2004.

Nies, B.L. *Eugenic Fantasies: Racial Ideology in the Literature and Popular Culture of the 1920's.* New York: Routledge, 2002.

Nietzsche, F. *Beyond Good and Evil,* trans. W. Kaufman, reprint edn. New York: Vintage Books, 1966.

———. *Twilight of the Idols/The Antichrist,* trans. R.J. Hollingdale, reprint edn. New York: Penguin Books, 1968.

———. *Thus Spoke Zarathustra,* trans. R.J. Hollingdale, reprint edn. London: Penguin Books, 1969.

Noakes, J. and Pridham, G. (eds). *Nazism 1919–1945: A History in Documents and Eyewitness Accounts,* vol. II: *Foreign Policy, War and Racial Extermination.* New York: Schocken Books, 1988.

Noël, L. *Intolerance: A General Survey,* trans. A. Bennett. Montreal and Kingston: McGill-Queen's University Press, 1994.

O'Brien, G.V. and Molinari, A. 'Religious metaphors as a justification for eugenic control: An historical analysis', in D. Schumm and M. Stoltzfus (eds.), *Disability in Judaism, Christianity and Islam: Sacred Texts, Historical Traditions and Social Analysis.* New York: Palgrave Macmillan, 2011, pp. 141–65.

Olby, R. *Origins of Mendelism.* Chicago: University of Chicago Press, 1985.

Oplinger, J. *The Politics of Demonology.* Selingsgrove: Sesquehanna University Press, 1990.

Parens, E. and Asch, A. (eds.). *Prenatal Testing and Disability Rights.* Washington, DC: Georgetown University Press, 2000.

Parker, R.A. *A Yankee Saint.* New York: G.P. Putnam's Sons, 1935.

Paul, J. 'State eugenic sterilization history: A brief overview', in J. Robitscher (ed.), *Eugenic Sterilization.* Springfield, IL: Charles C. Thomas, 1973, pp. 25–40.

Peel, J.D.Y. *Herbert Spencer: The Evolution of a Sociologist.* New York: Basic Books, Inc., 1971.

Pernick, M.S. *The Black Stork: Eugenics and the Death of 'Defective' Babies in American Medicine and Motion Pictures since 1915*. New York: Oxford University Press, 1996.

Peterson, J. *Early Conceptions and Tests of the Intelligence*. Westport, CT: Greenwood Press, 1969.

Pilcher, F.H. 'Superintendent's report', in *Seventh Biennial Report of the Superintendent, Kansas Asylum for Idiotic and Imbecile Youth at Winfield*. Topeka: Press of the Hamilton Printing Company, 1894, pp. 7–8.

Plato, *The Republic*, trans. D. Lee, reprint edn. Harmondsworth, Middlesex: Penguin Books, Ltd., 1986.

Poliakov, L. *The Aryan Myth*, trans. E. Howard. New York: Basic Books, Inc., 1974

Popenoe, P. and Johnson, R.H. *Applied Eugenics*. New York: Macmillan Co., 1933.

Proctor, R.N. *Racial Hygiene: Medicine under the Nazis*. Cambridge, MA: Harvard University Press, 1988.

——. *The Nazi War on Cancer*. Princeton, NJ: Princeton University Press, 1999.

Rafter, N.H. *White Trash: The Eugenic Family Studies 1877–1919*. Boston: Northeastern University Press, 1988.

Reilly, P.R. *The Surgical Solution: A History of Involuntary Sterilization in the United States*. Baltimore: Johns Hopkins University Press, 1991.

Rivera, G. *Willowbrook*. New York: Random House, 1972.

Roberts, P. *The New Immigration*. New York: Macmillan Company, 1914.

Robertson, C.N. *Oneida Community*. Syracuse: Syracuse University Press, 1970.

Rosen, C. *Preaching Eugenics: Religious Leaders and the American Eugenics Movement*. Oxford: Oxford University Press, 2004.

Sanford, N. and Comstock, C. (eds.). *Sanctions for Evil*. San Francisco: Jossey-Bass, Inc., 1971.

Sanger, M. *Woman and the New Race*. New York: Blue Ribbon Books, 1920.

——. *The Pivot of Civilization*. New York: Brentano's Publishers, 1922.

Sax, B. *Animals in the Third Reich: Pets, Scapegoats, and the Holocaust*. New York: Continuum International Publishing Group, Inc., 2000.

Saxton, M. 'Why members of the disability community oppose prenatal diagnosis and selective abortion', in Parens and Asch (eds.), *Prenatal Testing and Disability Rights*, pp. 147–64.

Scheerenberger, R.C. *A History of Mental Retardation*. Baltimore: Paul Brooks Publishing, 1983.

Scheinfeld, A. *You and Heredity*. New York: Frederick A. Stokes Co., 1939.

Schön, D.A. 'Generative metaphor: A perspective on problem-setting in social policy', in A. Ortony (ed.), *Metaphor and Thought*. New York: Cambridge University Press, 1979, pp. 254–83.

Selden, S. *Inheriting Shame: The Story of Eugenics and Racism in America*. New York: Teachers College, 1999.

Selzer, M. (ed.). *Kike: A Documentary History of Anti-Semitism in America*. New York: World Publishing, 1972.

Sereny, G. *Into that Darkness: From Mercy Killing to Mass Murder*. London: Andre Deutsch, 1974.

Shannon, T.W. *Nature's Secrets Revealed*, 3rd edn. Marietta, OH: S.A. Mullikin Company, 1915.

Shaw, B. *Man and Superman*, reprint edn. Baltimore: Penguin Books, 1952.

Shockley, W. 'Eugenic, or anti-dysgenic, thinking exercises', in R. Pearson (ed.), *Shockley on Eugenics and Race: The Application of Science to the Solution of Human Problems*, reprint edn. Washington, DC: Scott-Townsend Publishers, 1992, pp. 210–11.

Singer, P. *Animal Liberation: A New Ethics for Our Treatment of Animals*. New York: Avon Books, 1975.

——. 'All animals are equal', in T. Regan and P. Singer (eds.), *Animal Rights and Human Obligations*, reprint edn. Englewood Cliffs, NJ: Prentice Hall, 1989, pp. 73–83.

Skultans, V. *Madness and Morals: Ideas on Insanity in the Nineteenth Century*. London: Routledge & Kegan Paul, 1975.

Smith, J.D. *Minds Made Feeble: The Myth and Legacy of the Kallikaks*. Austin, TX: Pro-Ed, 1985.

—— and Nelson, K.R. *The Sterilization of Carrie Buck*. Far Hills, NJ: New Horizon Press, 1989.

Sontag, S. *Illness as Metaphor and AIDS and its Metaphors*. New York: Anchor Books, 1990.

Spencer, H. *Social Statics*, abridged and rev. version. New York: D. Appleton and Co., 1893.

——. *The Study of Sociology*. New York: D. Appleton and Company, 1904.

Spiro, J.P. *Defending the Master Race: Conservation, Eugenics, and the Legacy of Madison Grant*. Burlington, VT: University of Vermont Press, 2009.

Stoddard, L. *The Rising Tide of Color against White World-Supremacy*. New York: Charles Scribner's Sons, 1922.

——. *The Revolt against Civilization: The Menace of the Under Man*. New York: Charles Scribner's Sons, 1923.

——. *Racial Realities in Europe*. New York: Charles Scribner's Sons, 1925.

——. *Into the Darkness: Nazi Germany Today*. New York: Duell, Sloan & Pearce, Inc., 1940.

Szasz, T. *The Manufacture of Madness: A Comparative Study of the Inquisition and the Mental Health Movement*. New York: Harper and Row, 1970.

Talbot, E.S. *Degeneracy: Its Causes, Signs, and Results*, reprint edn. New York: Garland Publishing, Inc., 1984.

Taylor, F.W. *Scientific Management*, reprint edn. (New York: Harper & Brothers, 1947.

Thomson, R.G. 'Seeing the disabled: Visual rhetorics of disability in popular photography', in P.K. Longmore and L. Umansky (eds.), *The New Disability History*. New York: New York University Press, 2001, pp. 335–74.

Thorndike, L. *A History of Magic and Experimental Science*, vol. VIII, reprint edn. New York: Columbia University Press, 1964.

Tooley, M. *Abortion and Infanticide*. Oxford: Clarendon Press, 1983.

Trent, J.W., Jr. *Inventing the Feeble Mind: A History of Mental Retardation in the United States.* Berkeley: University of California Press, 1994.

Tucker, W.H. *The Science and Politics of Racial Research.* Urbana: University of Illinois Press, 1996.

Von Maltitz, H. *The Evolution of Hitler's Germany.* New York: McGraw-Hill Book Company, 1973.

Warne, F.J. *The Immigrant Invasion,* reprint edn. New York: American Immigration Library, 1971.

Weindling, P. *Health, Race and German Politics between National Unification and Naziism, 1870–1945.* Cambridge: Cambridge University Press, 1989.

——. *Epidemics and Genocide in Eastern Europe, 1890–1945.* Oxford: Oxford University Press, 2000.

Weir, R.F. *Selective Nontreatment of Handicapped Newborns,* New York: Oxford University Press, 1984.

Weiss, F.F. *The Sieve.* Boston: Page Co., 1921.

Wertham, F. *A Sign for Cain: An Exploration of Human Violence.* New York: Macmillan Co., 1966.

West, R. *Pickled Punks and Girlie Shows: A Life Spent on the Midways of America.* Atglen, PA: Schiffer Publishing, 2011.

Whetham, W. and Whetham, C. *The Family and the Nation: A Study in Natural Inheritance and Social Responsibility.* London: Longmans, Green, and Co., 1909.

Whitney, L.F. *The Source of Crime.* Reprinted from *Christian Work Magazine* by the American Eugenics Society, Inc. (1926).

——. *The Case for Sterilization.* New York: Frederick A. Stokes Co., 1934.

Wiggam, A.E. *The New Decalogue of Science.* Indianapolis: Bobbs-Merrill Company, 1923.

——. *The Fruit of the Family Tree.* Indianapolis: Bobbs-Merrill Company, 1924.

——. *The Next Age of Man.* Indianapolis: Bobbs-Merrill Company, 1927.

Wolfensberger, W. *The Principle of Normalization in Human Services.* Toronto: National Institute on Mental Retardation, 1972.

——. *The New Genocide of Handicapped and Afflicted People,* rev. edn. Syracuse, NY: Author, 1992.

Yukins, E. 'Feeble-minded white women and the spectre of proliferating perversity in American eugenics narratives', in L.A. Cuddy and C.M. Roche (eds.), *Evolution and Eugenics in American Literature and Culture, 1880–1940: Essays on Ideological Conflict and Complicity.* Lewisburg, PA: Bucknell University Press, 2003, pp. 164–86.

Zenderland, L. *Measuring Minds: Henry Herbert Goddard and the Origins of American Intelligence Testing.* Cambridge: Cambridge University Press, 1998.

Ziemer, G. *Education for Death: The Making of the Nazi.* London: Oxford University Press, 1941.

Conference and association proceedings and government documents

Bancroft, M. 'Classification of the mentally deficient', in *Proceedings of the National Conference on Charities and Correction*. Boston: Geo. H. Ellis, 1901, pp. 191–9.

Barr, M.W. 'The imbecile and epileptic *versus* the tax-payer and the community', in *Proceedings of the National Conference on Charities and Correction*. Boston: Geo. H. Ellis, 1902, pp. 161–5.

——. 'The prevention of mental defect, the duty of the hour', in *Proceedings of the National Conference on Charities and Correction*. Chicago: Hildmann Printing Co., 1915, pp. 361–7.

Broomall, J.M. 'The helpless classes', in *Proceedings of the Association of Medical Officers of American Institutions for Idiotic and Feeble-Minded Persons*. New York: Johnson Reprint Company Limited, 1887–95, pp. 38–41.

Buck v. Bell, 143 Va. Ct. App. Keyser-Doherty Printing Co., 1926, pp. 310–24.

Bullard, W.N. 'State care of high-grade imbecile girls', in *Proceedings of the National Conference on Charities and Correction*. Press of the Archer Printing Co., 1910, pp. 299–303.

Butler, A.W. 'The burden of feeble-mindedness', in *Proceedings of the National Conference on Charities and Correction*. Indianapolis: Press of Wm. B. Burford, 1907, pp. 1–10.

Carson, J.C. 'Prevention of feeble-mindedness from a moral and legal standpoint', in *Proceedings of the National Conference of Charities and Correction*. Boston: Geo. H. Ellis, 1898, pp. 294–303.

Cole, L.J. 'The relation of philanthropy and medicine to race betterment', in *Proceedings of the First National Conference on Race Betterment*. Battle Creek, MI: Race Betterment Foundation, 1914, pp. 494–508.

Congressional Record, Washington, DC: U.S. Government Printing Office, 18 February 1942, pp. 1419–20; 26 February 1942, pp. 1682–3.

Davenport, C.B. 'Eugenics and charity', in *Proceedings of the National Conference on Charities and Correction*. Fort Wayne, IN: Fort Wayne Printing Company, 1912, pp. 280–2.

——. 'Marriage laws and customs', in *Problems in Eugenics: Papers Communicated to the First International Eugenics Congress*. London: Eugenics Education Society, 1912, pp. 151–5.

——. 'Field work an indispensable aid to state care of the socially inadequate', in *Proceedings of the National Conference on Charities and Correction*. Chicago: Hildemann Printing Co., 1915, pp. 312–15.

——. 'Presidential address: The development of eugenics', in *A Decade of Progress in Eugenics: Scientific Papers of the Third International Congress of Eugenics*. Baltimore: Williams and Wilkins Company, 1934, pp. 17–22.

DeVilbiss, L.A. 'Better babies contests', in *Proceedings of the First National Conference on Race Betterment*. Battle Creek, MI: Race Betterment Foundation, 1914, pp. 554–5.

'Discussion on provision for the feeble-minded', in *Proceedings of the National Conference on Charities and Correction.* Boston: Geo. H. Ellis, 1888, pp. 395–402.

Dugdale, R.L. 'Hereditary pauperism', in *Proceedings of the Conference of Charities.* Boston: A. Williams & Co., 1877, pp. 81–99.

Eighteenth Biennial Report of the State Home for Feeble-Minded, Winfield, Kansas. Topeka: Kansas State Printing Plant, 1916.

Estabrook, A.H. 'The Tribe of Ishmael', in *Eugenics, Genetics and the Family*, vol. I: *Scientific Papers of the Second International Congress of Eugenics.* Baltimore: Williams & Wilkins Company, 1923, pp. 398–404.

Europe as an Emigrant-Exporting Continent and the United States as an Immigrant Receiving Nation. U.S. House of Representatives, Committee on Immigration and Naturalization. Testimony of Harry H. Laughlin, 8 March 1924, pp. 1231–318.

Fernald, W.E. 'Care of the feeble-minded', in *Proceedings of the National Conference on Charities and Correction.* Press of Fred J. Heer, 1904, pp. 380–90.

——. 'What is practical in the way of prevention of mental defect?', in *Proceedings of the National Conference on Charities and Correction.* Chicago: Hildemann Printing Co., 1915, pp. 289–307.

Fisher, I. 'Public health as a social movement', in *Proceedings of the National Conference of Social Work.* Chicago: National Conference of Social Work, 1917, pp. 183–93.

Gilman, R. 'Better babies', in *Proceedings of the First National Conference on Race Betterment.* Battle Creek, MI: Race Betterment Foundation, 1914, pp. 272–8.

Guyer, M.F. 'Sterilization', in *Proceedings of the Wisconsin Conference on Charities and Corrections.* Madison: Bobbs-Merrill Company, 1913, pp. 33–60.

Hart, H.H. 'Segregation', in *Proceedings of the First National Conference on Race Betterment.* Battle Creek, MI: Race Betterment Foundation, 1914, pp. 403–10.

Hickson, W.J. 'The criminal in everyday life', in *Proceedings of the Third National Conference on Race Betterment.* Battle Creek, MI: Race Betterment Foundation, 1928, pp. 148–53.

Hinshaw, T.E. 'Physician's report', in *Twenty-Second Biennial Report of the State Training School, Winfield Kansas.* Topeka: Kansas State Printing Plant, 1924, p. 19.

Jennings, H.S. 'Health progress and race progress: Are they compatible?', in *American Association for the Study of the Feebleminded: Proceedings and Addresses of the Fifty-First Annual Session.* American Association for the Study of the Feebleminded, 1927, pp. 232–42.

Johnson, A. 'Permanent custodial care: Report of Committee on the Care of the Feeble Minded', in *Proceedings of the National Conference on Charities and Correction.* Boston: Geo. H. Ellis, 1896, pp. 207–19.

——. 'Custodial care', in *Proceedings of the National Conference of Charities and Correction.* Fort Wayne, IN: Press of Fort Wayne Printing Co., 1908, pp. 333–6.

Johnstone, E.R. 'Practical provision for the mentally deficient', in *Proceedings of the National Conference of Charities and Correction.* Fort Wayne, IN: Press of Fort Wayne Printing Co., 1908, pp. 316–25.

——. 'Committee report: Stimulating public interest in the feeble-minded', in

Proceedings of the National Conference of Charities and Correction. Chicago: Hildmann Printing Co., 1916, pp. 205–15.

Keene, G.F. 'The genesis of the defective', in *Proceedings of the National Conference on Charities and Correction.* Press of Fred J. Heer, 1904, pp. 407–18.

Kellogg, J.H. 'Eugenics and immigration: Needed – a new human race', in *Proceedings of the First National Conference on Race Betterment.* Battle Creek, MI: Race Betterment Foundation, 1914, pp. 431–42.

——. 'Eugenics Registry Office', in *Proceedings of the First National Conference on Race Betterment.* Battle Creek, MI: Race Betterment Foundation, 1914, pp. 564–5.

Knight, G.H. 'Prevention from a legal and moral standpoint', in *Proceedings of the National Conference on Charities and Correction.* Boston: Geo. H. Ellis, 1898, pp. 304–8.

Little, C.C. 'President's address: Shall we live longer and should we?', in *Proceedings of the Third Race Betterment Conference.* Battle Creek, MI: Race Betterment Foundation, 1928, pp. 5–19.

McDougall, W. 'A national fund for a new plan of remuneration as a eugenic measure', in *Second International Congress of Eugenics,* vol. II. Baltimore: Williams & Wilkins Company, 1923, pp. 62–3.

MacMurchy, H. 'The relation of feeble-mindedness to other social problems', in *Proceedings of the National Conference on Charities and Correction.* Chicago: Hildmann Printing Co., 1916, pp. 229–35.

Martin, W.F. 'Better babies contest', in *Proceedings of the First National Conference on Race Betterment.* Battle Creek, MI: Race Betterment Foundation, 1914, pp. 554–5.

Mastin, J.T. 'The new colony plan for the feeble-minded', in *Proceedings of the National Conference on Charities and Correction.* Chicago: Hildmann Printing Co., 1916, pp. 239–50.

Mott, A.J. 'The education and custody of the imbecile', in *Proceedings of the National Conference on Charities and Correction.* Boston: Press of Geo. H. Ellis, 1894, pp. 168–79.

Murdoch, J.M. 'Quarantine mental defectives', in *Proceedings of the National Conference on Charities and Correction.* Fort Wayne, IN: Fort Wayne Printing Co., 1909, pp. 64–7.

Nazi Conspiracy and Aggression, vol. V. Office of United States Chief of Counsel for Prosecution of Axis Criminality. Washington, DC: United States Government Printing Office, 1947.

Olson, Judge H. 'The menace of the half-man', in *Proceedings of the Third Race Betterment Conference.* Battle Creek, MI: Race Betterment Foundation, 1928, pp. 122–47.

Plecker, W.A. 'Virginia's effort to preserve racial integrity', in *A Decade of Progress in Eugenics: Scientific Papers of the Third International Congress of Eugenics.* Baltimore: Williams and Wilkens Co., 1934, pp. 105–12.

Robie, T.R. 'Selective sterilization for race culture', in *A Decade of Progress in Eugenics: Scientific Papers of the Third International Congress of Eugenics.* Baltimore: Williams and Wilkens Co., 1934, pp. 201–9.

Rogers, A.C. 'Colonizing the feeble-minded', in *Proceedings of the National Conference on Charities and Correction*. Press of Fred J. Heer, 1903, pp. 254–8.

Sanborn, B.T. 'The care of the feeble-minded', in *Proceedings of the National Conference on Charities and Correction*. Press of Fred J. Heer, 1904, pp. 401–7.

Southard, E.E. 'The feeble-minded as subjects of research in efficiency', in *Proceedings of the National Conference on Charities and Correction*. Chicago: Hildemann Printing Co., 1915, pp. 315–19.

Stern, L. 'Heredity and environment: The Bilder clan', in *Proceedings of the National Conference of Social Work*. Chicago: University of Chicago Press, 1922, pp. 179–89.

Sumner, Rev. W.T. 'The health certificate: A safeguard against vicious selection in marriage', in *Proceedings of the First National Conference on Race Betterment*. Battle Creek, MI: Race Betterment Foundation, 1914, pp. 509–12.

Taft, J. 'Supervision of the feebleminded in the community', in *Proceedings of the National Conference of Social Work*. Chicago: Rogers & Hall Co., 1918, pp. 543–50.

United States Department of Energy. *Advisory Committee on Human Radiation Experiments: Final Report*, Washington, DC: U.S. Government Printing Office, 1995.

Van Wagenen, B. 'The eugenic problem', in *Proceedings of the National Conference of Charities and Correction*. Fort Wayne, IN: Fort Wayne Printing Company, 1912, pp. 275–9.

Ward, R.D. 'Race betterment and our immigration laws', in *Proceedings of the First Race Betterment Conference*. Battle Creek, MI: Race Betterment Foundation, 1914, pp. 542–6.

Warthin, A.S. 'A biologic philosophy or religion a necessary foundation for race betterment', in *Proceedings of the Third Race Betterment Conference*. Battle Creek, MI: Race Betterment Foundation, 1928, pp. 86–90.

Weidensall, J. 'The mentality of the unmarried mother', in *Proceedings of the National Conference of Social Work*. Chicago: National Conference of Social Work, 1917, pp. 287–94.

Wells, K.G. 'State regulation of marriage', in *Proceedings of the National Conference of Charities and Correction*, Boston: Geo. H. Ellis, 1897, pp. 302–8.

Whitney, E.A. and Shick, M.M. 'Some results of selective sterilization', in *American Association for the Study of the Feebleminded: Proceedings and Addresses of the Fifty-Fifth Annual Session*. American Association for the Study of the Feebleminded, 1931, pp. 330–38.

Wilmarth, A.W. 'Report of Committee on Feeble-Minded and Epileptic', in *Proceedings of the National Conference of Charities and Correction*. Boston: Geo. H. Ellis, 1902, pp. 152–61.

Wright, A.O. 'The defective classes', in *Proceedings of the National Conference on Charities and Correction*. Boston: Geo. H. Ellis, 1891, pp. 222–9.

Journal and newspaper articles

Allbritton, D.W. 'When metaphors function as schemas: Some cognitive effects of conceptual metaphors', *Metaphor and Symbolic Activity* 10 (1995), 33–46.

Allen, G.E. 'Science misapplied: The eugenic age revisited', *Technology Review* 99:6 (1996), 23–31.

Altman, R. 'Selection from the skies', (translation), *Living Age* 357:4477 (1939), 132–5.

Annas, G.J. 'Reframing the debate on health care reform by replacing our metaphors', *New England Journal of Medicine* 332 (1995), 744–7.

'Ape-footed man', *Eugenics* 1:2 (1928), 27.

Armstrong, C. 'The moron menace', *Birth Control Review* 22:5 (1938), 52–3.

'Autopsy Puts boy in class of defectives', *New York Times* (18 November 1915), 1.

Baldwin, B.T. 'The psychology of mental deficiency', *Popular Science Monthly* 79 (1911), 82–93.

Barr, M.W. 'President's annual address', *Journal of Psycho-Asthenics* 2 (1897), 1–13.

——. 'Defective children: Their needs and their rights', *International Journal of Ethics* 8 (1898), 481–90.

——. 'Mental defectives and the social welfare', *Popular Science Monthly* 54 (1899), 746–59.

Batten, S.Z. 'The redemption of the unfit', *American Journal of Sociology* 14 (1908), 233–60.

Bell, A.G. 'How to improve the race', *Journal of Heredity* 5:1 (1914), 1–7.

Bicknell, E.P. 'Custodial care of the adult feeble-minded', *Charities Review* 5 (November 1895–June 1896), 76–88.

Binding, K. and Hoche, A. 'Permitting the destruction of unworthy life: Its extent and form' (1920), trans. W.E. Wright, *Issues in Law and Medicine* 8 (1992), 231–65.

'"Biological Purge" is urged by Hooton', *New York Times* (21 February 1937), section II, 1–2.

'Birth control is peril to race, says Osborn', *New York Times* (23 August 1932), 1, 16.

Blount, A. 'Eugenics in relation to birth control', *Birth Control Review* 2:1 (1918), 7, 15.

Bock, G. 'Racism and sexism in Nazi Germany: Motherhood, compulsory sterilization, and the state', *Signs* 8 (1983), 400–21.

Bogdan, R. 'Exhibiting mentally retarded people for amusement and profit, 1850–1940', *American Journal of Mental Deficiency* 91 (1986), 120–6.

Brave, R. and Sylva, K. 'Exhibiting eugenics: Response and resistance to a hidden history', *Public Historian* 29:3 (2007), 33–51.

Bryce, P.H. 'Feeblemindedness and social environment', *American Journal of Public Health* 8 (1918), 656–60.

Buell, R.L. 'The development of anti-Japanese agitation in the United States, II', *Political Science Quarterly* 38 (1923), 57–81.

Burke, C.S. and Castaneda, C.J. 'The public and private history of eugenics: An introduction', *Public Historian* 29:3 (2007), 5–17.

Butler, A.W. 'A notable factor of social degeneracy', *Indiana Bulletin* (December 1901), 17–25.

Campbell, C. 'Praise for Nazis', *Time* (9 September 1935), 20–1.

Cannon, C.J. 'Selecting citizens', *North American Review* 217 (1923), 325–33.

'Case for sterilization', *Living Age* 357 (1939), 135–7.

'Christ was an Aryan', *Living Age* 352 (1937), 318–21.

Clark, L.P. 'Idiocy and laboratory research', *Survey* 27 (1912), 1857–60.

Cockburn, A. 'Beat the devil', *Nation* (23 November 1992), 618–19.

——. 'Social cleansing', *New Statesman and Society* (August 1994), 16–18.

Cohen, C.B. 'The Nazi analogy in bioethics' (commentary), *Hastings Center Report* 18:5 (1988), 32–3.

Cole, L.J. 'Biological eugenics', *Journal of Heredity* 5 (1914), 305–12.

'Committee on Cooperation with Clergymen', *Eugenical News* 10:5 (1925), 68.

Cox, I.W. 'The folly of human sterilization', *Scientific American* 151 (1934), 188–90.

Crook, P. 'American eugenics and the Nazis: Recent historiography', *European Legacy* 7 (2002), 363–81.

Daggett, M.P. 'Women: Building a better race', *World's Work* 25 (1912), 229–34.

Darlington, T. 'The medico-economic aspect of the immigration problem', *North American Review* 183 (1906), 1262–71.

Davenport, C.B. 'Report of Committee on Eugenics', *American Breeders Magazine* 1:2 (1910), 126–9.

——. 'The origin and control of mental defectiveness', *Popular Science Monthly* 80 (1912), 87–90.

——. 'The Nams: The feeble-minded as country dwellers', *Survey* 27 (1912), 1844–45.

——. 'Importance of heredity to the state', *Indiana Bulletin* (September 1913), 394–413.

——. 'Research in eugenics', *Science* 54 (1921), 391–6.

Davenport, G.C. 'Hereditary crime', *American Journal of Sociology* 13 (November 1907), 402–9.

Davis, J.J. 'Jail – or a passport: Some facts and views of immigration', *Saturday Evening Post* (1 December 1923), 23, 134, 137.

Davis, K.B. 'Feeble-minded women in reformatory institutions', *Survey* 27 (1912), 1849–51.

'Doctor to let patient's baby defective die', *Chicago Tribune* (17 November 1915), 1.

Dodge, E. 'Bettering the birthrates', *Journal of Heredity* 15:3 (1924), 113–18.

'Does the world need more morons?', *Eugenics* 2:4 (1929), 20–2.

Drimmer, J.C. 'Cripples, overcomers, and civil rights: Tracing the evolution of federal legislation and social policy for people with disabilities', *UCLA Law Review* 40 (1993), 1341–410.

Dudziak, M.L. 'Oliver Wendell Holmes as a eugenic reformer: Rhetoric in the writing of constitutional law', *Iowa Law Review* 71 (1986), 833–67.

'Echoes of the Eugenics Congress', *Journal of Heredity* 23 (1932), 385–6.

Elks, M.A. 'The "lethal chamber": Further evidence for the euthanasia option', *Mental Retardation* 31 (1993), 201–7.

Ellis, W.T. 'Americans on guard', *Saturday Evening Post* (25 August 1923), 23, 80, 83, 86.

Ellwood, W.N. 'Declaring war on the home front: Metaphor, presidents, and the war on drugs', *Metaphor and Symbolic Activity* 10:2 (1995), 93–114.

Emerson, H. 'Eugenics in relation to medicine', *Journal of Heredity* 30 (1939), 553–6.

Enderis, G. 'Reich takes over rights of states', *New York Times* (31 January 1934), 13.

Estabrook, A.H. 'A two-family apartment', *Survey* 29 (1913), 853–4.

'Eugenical sterilization in Germany', *Eugenical News* 18:5 (1933), 89–94.

'Eugenics and democracy: A paradox', *Journal of Heredity* 23:5 (1932), 221–2.

'Eugenics supported by the church', *Current Literature* 52 (1912), 565–6.

Evans, S.W. 'Eugenics on parade', *Eugenics* 3:10 (1930), 390–4.

Fairchild, H.P. 'From dysgenic to eugenic birth control', *Birth Control Review* 2:7 (1935), 2–3.

'Feeble minded boys committed under new law', *Chicago Tribune* (19 November 1915), 5.

Fernald, W.E. 'The imbecile with criminal instincts', *Journal of Psycho-Asthenics* 14 (1909), 16–36.

———. 'The burden of feeble-mindedness', *Journal of Psycho-Asthenics* 17 (1912), 87–99.

———. 'The feeble-minded', *Educational Review* 54 (1917), 118–27.

Fisher, I. 'Impending problems of eugenics', *Scientific Monthly* 13 (1921), 214–31.

Frankel, C. 'The specter of eugenics', *Commentary* 57 (March 1974), 25–33.

Frazer, E. 'Our foreign cities: Chicago', *Saturday Evening Post* (25 August 1923), 14.

Frick, W. 'German population and race politics', trans. A. Hellmer, *Eugenical News* 19:2 (1934), 33–8.

Frost, W.A. 'A race of human thoroughbreds: An authorized interview with Alexander Graham Bell', *World's Work* 27 (1913), 176–82.

'The future of America: A biological forecast', *Harpers Magazine* 156 (1928), 529–39.

Gallagher, H.G. '"Slapping up spastics": The persistence of social attitudes toward people with disabilities', *Issues in Law & Medicine* 10 (1995), 401–14.

Galton, F. 'Eugenics: Its definition, scope, and aims', *American Journal of Sociology* 10 (1904), 1–25 (discussion included).

Gamble, C.J. 'Eugenic sterilization in the United States', *Eugenical News* 34: 1–2 (1949), 1–5.

Gardner, J.M. 'Contribution of the German cinema to the Nazi euthanasia program', *Mental Retardation* 20 (1982), 174–5.

Gelb, S.A. 'The beast in man: Degeneration and mental retardation, 1900–1920', *Mental Retardation* 33 (1995), 1–9.

Gerdtz, J., 'Disability and euthanasia: The case of Helen Keller and the Bollinger baby', *Life and Learning* 16 (2006), 491–500.

Goddard, H.H. 'Psychological work among the feeble-minded', *Journal of Psycho-Asthenics* 12 (1907), 18–30.

——. 'Four hundred feeble-minded children classified by the Binet method', *Journal of Psycho-Asthenics* 15 (1910), 17–30.

——. 'Wanted: A child to adapt', *Survey* 27 (1911), 1003–6.

——. 'The basis for state policy: Social investigation and prevention', *Survey* 27 (1912), 1852–4.

——. 'Sterilization and segregation', *Indiana Bulletin* (December 1912), 424–8.

——. 'The hereditary factor in feeble-mindedness', *Institution Quarterly* 4:2 (1913), 9–11.

Gosney, E.S. 'Eugenic sterilization: Human betterment demands it', *Scientific American* 151 (1934), 18–19, 52–3.

'Guarding the gates against undesirables', *Current Opinion* 76 (1924), 400–1.

Hanauske-Able, H.M. 'From Nazi holocaust to nuclear holocaust: A lesson to learn?', *Lancet* 2:8501 (1986), 271–3.

Harding, T.S. 'Are we breeding weaklings?', *American Journal of Sociology* 42 (1936), 672–81.

Hardt, H.G. 'Care of feeble-minded women', *Institution Quarterly* 3:1 (1912), 179–86.

Harrington, A. 'Metaphoric connections: Holistic science in the shadow of the Third Reich', *Social Research* 62 (1995), 357–85.

Haslam, N. 'Dehumanization: An integrative review', *Personality and Social Psychology Review* 10 (2006), 252–64.

Henley, M. 'The creation and perpetuation of the mother/body myth: Judicial and legislative enlistment of Norplant', *Buffalo Law Review* 41 (1993), 734–59.

Hollander, R. 'Euthanasia and mental retardation: Thinking the unthinkable', *Mental Retardation* 27 (1989), 53–62.

Holmes, A. 'Eugenics', *Institution Quarterly* 5:1 (1914), 151–61.

Holt, W.L. 'Economic factors in eugenics', *Popular Science Monthly* 83 (1913), 471–83.

'Hooton finds man reverting to ape', *New York Times* (4 December 1937), 27.

Humphrey, S. 'Parenthood and social conscience', *Forum* 49 (1913), 457–64.

——. 'Men and half-men', *Scribners Magazine* 73 (1923), 284–7.

'Husbanding the nation's manhood', *World's Work* 20 (1910), 13470–1.

'Immigration checks the native birth rate', *World's Work* 46 (1923), 121–2.

'Intelligence wane seen by Dr. Hooton', *New York Times* (18 February 1937), 1.

Irwin, E.A. 'Fragments of humanity', *Survey* (2 March 1912), 1875.

'Is serum hepatitis only a special type of infectious hepatitis?', *Journal of the American Medical Association* 200 (1967), 136–7.

Jenish, D. 'What would you do?', *Maclean's* 107:48 (1994), 16–24.

Johnson, A. 'The case of the nation *vs.* the feebleminded', *Survey* 34 (1915), 136–7.

——. 'Children who never grow up: Some adventures among the feeble-minded', *Survey* 49 (1922–23), 310–16, 340.

——. 'Mixed crops: Some more adventures among the feeble-minded', *Survey* 49 (1922–23), 439–44, 465–6.

Johnson, E.H. 'Feeble-minded as city dwellers', *Survey* 27 (1912), 1840–3.

'The Jukes in 1915', *Journal of Heredity* 7 (1916), 469–74.

Keller, H. 'Physicians' juries for defective babies' (letter to the editor), *New Republic* (18 December 1915), 173.

Kempton, J.H. 'Sterilization for ten million Americans' (book review), *Journal of Heredity* 25 (1934), 415–18.

Kennedy, A.C. 'Eugenics, "degenerate girls", and social workers during the Progressive Era', *Affilia: Journal of Women and Social Work* 23 (2008), 22–37.

Kennedy, F. 'Euthanasia: To be or not to be', *Colliers* 103 (20 May 1939), 15–16.

Kirkbride, F.B. 'The right to be well-born', *Survey* 27 (1912), 1838–9.

Kirkbride, M.B. 'The army of sorrow', *Survey* 26 (1911), 228.

Kite, E.S. 'Two brothers', *Survey* 27 (1912), 1861–4.

——. 'Unto the third generation', *Survey* 28 (1912), 789–91.

——. 'Mental defect as found by the field-worker', *Journal of Psycho-Asthenics* 17 (1913), 145–54.

——. 'The "Piney's"', *Survey* 31 (1913), 9–13, 38–40.

Knox, H.A. 'Tests for mental defects', *Journal of Heredity* 5 (1914), 122–30.

Krohn, F. 'Military metaphors', *Et Cetera: A Review of General Semantics* 44 (1987), 141–5.

Krugman, S., Giles, J., and Hammond, J. 'Infectious hepatitis: Evidence for two distinctive clinical, epidemiological and immunological types of infection', *Journal of the American Medical Association* 200 (1967), 95–103.

Lakoff, G. 'Metaphor, morality, and politics, or, Why conservatives have left liberals in the dust', *Social Research* 62 (1995), 177–213.

Landman, J.H. 'Race betterment by human sterilization', *Scientific American* 150 (1934), 292–5.

Laughlin, H.H. 'Report on the organization and the first eight months' work of the Eugenics Record Office', *American Breeders Magazine* 2:2 (1911), 107–12.

——. 'An account of the work of the Eugenics Record Office', *American Breeders Magazine* 3:2 (1912), 119–23.

——. 'First Annual Conference of Eugenics Field Workers', *American Breeders Magazine* 3:4 (1912), 265–9.

——. 'The eugenical sterilization of the feeble-minded', *Journal of Psycho-Asthenics* 31 (1925), 210–18.

——. 'Further studies on the historical and legal development of eugenical sterilization in the United States', *Journal of Psycho-Asthenics* 41 (1936), 96–110.

——. Letter to Dr C. Schneider, 28 May 1936. Harry H. Laughlin Papers, Pectler Memorial Library, Truman State University.

LeBourdais, D.M. 'Purifying the human race', *North American Review* 238 (1934), 431–7.

Lennox, W.G. 'Should they live?', *American Scholar* 7 (1938), 454–66.

'Lets afflicted baby die', *The New York Times* (28 January 1918), 6.

Levine, D.N. 'The organism metaphor in sociology', *Social Research* 62 (1995), 239–65.

Lorimar, F. 'Eugenics and birth control', *Birth Control Review* 16:8 (1932), 229–31.

Lovett, L.L. '"Fitter families for future firesides": Florence Sherbon and popular eugenics', *Public Historian* 29:3 (2007), 69–85.

Lyons, A. 'Ungraded parents', *Education* 38 (1917), 338–40.

MacMurchy, H. 'The relation of feeble-mindedness to other social problems', *Journal of Psycho-Asthenics* 21 (1916), 58–63.

'Major Darwin predicts civilization's doom unless century brings wide eugenic reforms', *New York Times* (23 August 1932), 16.

'The menace of the feeble-minded', *Eugenical News* 11:2 (1926), 34–5.

Mencken, H.L. 'Utopia by sterilization', *American Mercury* 41 (1937), 399–408.

'Mercy death law ready for albany', *New York Times* (14 February 1939), 2.

'Minutes of the Association', *Journal of Psycho-Asthenics* 22 (1917), 20–37.

Mügge, M.A. 'Eugenics and the superman: A racial science, and a racial religion', *Eugenics Review* 1 (1909–10), 184–206.

Musolff, A. 'What role do metaphors play in racial prejudice? The function of anti-semitic imagery in Hitler's *Mein Kampf*, *Patterns of Prejudice* 41 (2007), 21–43.

'Nazified medicine', *New York Times* (6 December 1942), section IV, 11.

'The need for further study of the Piney families', *Eugenical News* 10:6 (1925), 77–8.

Nelkin, D. and Gilman, S.L. 'Placing blame for devastating disease', *Social Research* 55 (1988), 361–78.

'A new force in the war on feeble-mindedness', *Survey* 29 (1913), 487–9.

'New German etymology for eugenics', *Eugenical News* 19:5 (1934), 125–6.

O'Brien, G.V. '"Protecting the social body: Use of the organism metaphor in fighting the "menace of the feeble-minded"', *Mental Retardation* 37 (1999), 188–200.

———. 'Indigestible food, conquering hordes, and waste materials: Metaphors of immigrants and the early immigration restriction debate in the U.S.', *Metaphor and Symbol* 18 (2003), 33–47.

———. 'Speciesism revisited: The potential for reversibility of the argument from marginal cases (AMC)', *Social Work* 48 (2003), 331–7.

———. 'Metaphors and the pejorative framing of marginalized groups: Implications for social work education', *Journal of Social Work Education* 45 (2009), 29–46.

———. 'Social justice implications of the organism metaphor', *Journal of Sociology and Social Welfare* 37 (2010), 95–113.

———. 'Anchors on the ship of progress and weeds in the human garden: Objectivist rhetoric in American eugenic writings', *Disability Studies Quarterly* 31:3 (2011), www.dsq-sds.org, accessed August 2011.

———. 'Eugenics, genetics and the minority group model of disabilities: Implications for social work advocacy', *Social Work* 56 (2011), 347–54.

——— and Bundy, M. '"Reaching beyond the 'moron" Eugenic control of secondary disability groups', *Journal of Sociology and Social Welfare* 36 (2009), 153–71.

Offen, M.L. 'Dealing with "defectives": Foster Kennedy and William Lennox on Eugenics', *Neurology* 61 (2003), 668–3.

Paradise, V.I. 'Three per cent', *Harper's Monthly Magazine* 144 (1922), 505–14.

Park, Y. and Kemp, S.P. '"Little alien colonies": Representations of immigrants and their neighborhoods in social work discourse, 1875–1924', *Social Service Review* 80 (2006), 705–34.

Parker, G.H. 'The eugenics movement as a public service', *Science* 41 (1915), 342–7.

Peabody, J.B. 'Putting it up to philanthropy' (letter to the editor), *Survey* 29 (1912), 98–9.

Pearl, R. 'Biology and human progress', *Harper's Monthly Magazine* 172 (1935–6), 225–35.

Pernick, M.S. 'Contagion and culture', *American Literary History* 14 (2002), 858–65.

Peter, W.W. 'Germany's sterilization program', *American Journal of Public Health* 24 (1934), 187–91.

'Pictures the cure for legislative sloth', *Survey* 37 (1917), 725–6.

'The plea for immigrants a plea for inefficiency', *World's Work* 46 (1923), 122–3.

Popenoe, P. 'Birth control and eugenics', *Birth Control Review* 1:3 (1917), 6.

———. 'The German sterilization law', *Journal of Heredity* 25 (1934), 257–60.

———. 'The progress of eugenic sterilization', *Journal of Heredity* 25 (1934), 19–25.

———. 'Should bachelors and fathers get the same pay?', *Eugenical News* 28:4 (1943), 52.

Powlison, C.F. 'Behold a sower went forth to sow', *Birth Control Review* 16:1 (1932), 5–7.

Pringle, H.N. 'Carnival shows', *Light* 140 (1921), 23–4.

'Prizes for sermons on eugenics', *Eugenical News* 11:3 (1926), 48.

Reccord, A.P. 'A perfectly normal child', *Survey* 41 (1918), 381.

Reeves, H.T. 'The later years of a noted mental defective', *Journal of Psycho-Asthenics* 43 (1938), 194–200.

Rentoul, R.R. 'Proposed sterilization of certain mental degenerates', *American Journal of Sociology* 12 (1906), 319–27.

Risley, S.D. 'Is asexualization ever justifiable in the case of imbecile children?', *Journal of Psycho-Asthenics* 9 (1905), 92–8.

Ritvo, H. 'Border trouble: Shifting the line between people and other animals', *Social Research* 62 (1995), 481–500.

Robie, T. 'Towards race betterment', *Birth Control Review* 17:4 (1933), 93–5.

Robinson, C.H. 'Toward curbing differential births and lowering taxes: A plank or two for eugenic platforms', *Journal of Heredity* 29 (1938), 230–4.

———. 'Toward curbing differential births and lowering taxes, II: Eugenic custody for unfit breeders', *Journal of Heredity* 29 (1938), 260–4.

Roosevelt, T. 'Twisted eugenics', *American Motherhood* 38 (1914), 308–12.

Roper, A.G. 'Ancient eugenics', *Mankind Quarterly* 32 (1992), 383–418.

Ryan, P.J. '"Six blacks from home": Childhood, motherhood, and eugenics in America', *Journal of Policy History* 19 (2007), 253–81.

Ryder, D.W. 'The Japanese Bugaboo', *American Mercury* 3 (September 1924), 24–30.

Sanger, M. 'Birth control and racial betterment', *Birth Control Review* 3:2 (1919), 11–12.

Sanville, F.L. 'Social legislation in the Keystone State: A program in behalf of the mentally unfit', *Survey* 33 (1915), 667–70.

'"Saving Homo sapiens": Professor Hooton Sees hope only in applying eugenics', *New York Times* (28 February 1927), section XII, 8.

Schwartz, K. 'Nature's corrective principle in social evolution', *Journal of Psycho-Asthenics* 13 (1908), 74–90.

'Service from imbeciles', *Literary Digest* 53 (1916), 554–5.

Sessions, M.A. 'Feeble-minded in Ohio', *Journal of Heredity* 8 (1917), 291–7.

Shannon, T.W. 'Double standard and race degeneracy', *Light* 138 (March–April 1921), 35–9.

Shakespeare, T. 'Cultural representation for disabled people: Dustbins for disavowal?', *Disability & Society* 9 (1994), 283–99.

Sherbon, F.B. 'Eugenics and democracy: Are the two compatible?', *Eugenics* 2:9 (1929), 28–9.

Shipley, M. 'The sterilization of defectives', *American Mercury* 15 (1928), 454–7.

Slater, E. 'German eugenics in practice', *Eugenics Review* 27:4 (1936), 285–95.

Smith, J.D. 'Reflections on mental retardation and eugenics, old and new: Mensa and the Human Genome Project', *Mental Retardation* 32 (1994), 234–8.

'Sterilization law is termed humane', *New York Times* (22 January 1934), 6.

'Sterilize the feeble-minded? Pro and con', *Reader's Digest* 32 (May 1938), 97–103.

Stoddard, L. 'Worthwhile Americans', *Saturday Evening Post* 197 (17 January 1925), 23, 146–7, 149–50.

Storer, M. 'The defective delinquent girl', *Journal of Psycho-Asthenics* 19 (1914), 25–30.

Strother, F. 'The cause of crime: Defective brain', *World of Work* 48 (1924), 275–86.

Thomalia, C. 'The sterilization law in Germany', trans. A. Hellmer, *Eugenical News* 19:6 (1934), 137–40.

Thompson, C.B. 'Conservation of minds' (letter to the editor), *Survey* 38 (1917), 362.

Thurston, R. 'The Nazi war on medicine', *New Republic* 84 (4 December 1935), 100–2.

Trent, J.W., Jr. 'Defectives at the World's Fair: Constructing disability in 1904', *Remedial and Special Education* 19 (1998), 201–11.

'"The typhoon": A dramatization of the yellow peril', *Current Literature* 52 (1912), 567–73.

'U.S. Eugenicist hails Nazi racial policy', *New York Times* (29 August 1935), 5.

Van Wagenen, B. 'Surgical sterilization as a eugenic measure', *Journal of Psycho-Asthenics* 18 (1914), 185–96.

Voss, J.F., Kennet, J., Wiley, J., and Schooler, T.Y.E. 'Experts at debate: The use of metaphor in the U.S. Senate debate on the Gulf Crisis', *Metaphor and Symbolic Activity* 7 (1992), 197–214.

Wallin, W.E.W. 'A program for the state care of the feeble-minded and epileptic', *School and Society* 4 (11 November 1916), 723–31.

Ward, R.D. 'Natural eugenics in relation to immigration', *North American Review* 192 (1910), 56–67.

——. 'The crisis in our immigration policy', *Institution Quarterly* 4:2 (1913), 37–50.

——. 'Eugenic immigration', *American Breeders Magazine* 4:2 (1913), 96–102.

'Was the doctor right? Some independent opinions', *Independent* 85:3500 (1916), 23–27.

Weingartner, J. 'War against subhumans: Comparisons between the German war against the Soviet Union and the American war against Japan, 1941–1945', *Historian* 58 (1996), 557–73.

Whelpley, J.D. 'The overtaxed melting-pot', *Living Age* 281 (1914), 67–72.

Whitney, E.A. 'A hunt for society's danger spot', *Eugenics* 1:1 (1928), 25–30.

——. 'A plea for the control of feeble-mindedness', *Eugenics* 2:5 (1929), 12–13.

——. 'Selective sterilization' *Birth Control Review* 17:4 (1933), 85–7.

Wiggam, A.E. 'The rising tide of degeneracy: What everyone ought to know about eugenics', *World's Work* 53 (November 1926), 4–32.

Wolfensberger, W. 'The extermination of handicapped people in World War II Germany', *Mental Retardation* 19 (1981), 1–7.

Young, K. 'Intelligence tests of certain immigrant groups', *Scientific Monthly* 15 (1922), 417–34.

Zeleny, L.D. 'Feeble-mindedness and criminal conduct', *American Journal of Sociology* 38 (1933), 564–76.

Zuckier, H. 'The essential "other" and the Jew: From antisemitism to genocide', *Social Research* 63 (1996), 1110–52.

Index

Note: Literary works can be found under author's names

Agassiz, Louis 57
alarm movements, description 2, 24
  anti-African-American 31, 84, 106,
    162
  anti-Asian 2, 31, 44, 83–4, 106, 133,
    162
  anti-communist 2, 56, 84, 92, 162
  anti-immigrant 8–9, 31, 134, 140
  anti-Semitic 84, 106, 133–4, 162
alcoholic, moron as 116
Allbritton, David 19–20
Allen, Garland 168
altruistic metaphor 57, 107–8, 117–23
  euthanasia and 107–8, 122–3
  institutionalization and 118–19
  sterilization and 120–2
  unborn persons and 123
American Association for Study of the
  Feeble-minded 91
American eugenics movement 3–5,
  7–11, 149
American Eugenics Society 9, 111
anchor, weight or brake, moron as 140,
  142
anencephaly 169
animal or plant breeding, eugenics and 7,
  61, 135–7, 139
  see also Burbank, Luther
animal rights, eugenics and 71–2, 74
Annas, George 24
argument from marginal cases 74
Armstrong, Clairette 93
atavism 57–8

Baker, LaReine 114
  Race Improvement or Eugenics 114
Baldwin, Bird 145
Bancroft, Margaret 59
Barr, Martin 33–4, 40, 87–8, 113, 118,
  120, 138, 165
Bayle, François 60

behaviour modification 74
Bell, Alexander Graham 61, 162
Bernstein, Charles 40
better babies contests 10
  see also fitter families contests
Bethlam hospital 59
Bible, eugenics and the 109–11, 136
Bicknell, Earnest 165
Bilder clan 69
  see also eugenic family studies
Binding, Karl 65, 71, 122, 143
Binet, Alfred 64, 164
birth control see eugenic control methods
birth control movement 9, 96, 144–5
birth differential argument 33, 85, 94–6,
  145, 147
Blatt, Burton 21, 55, 75, 151, 166–7
blindness, eugenics and 165–6
blood, organism metaphor and 31, 34,
  36
Bogdan, Robert 59
Bollinger Baby 65, 69, 90, 112, 122, 143,
  147, 166
Bonnaterre, Pierre-Joseph 60
Braille, Louis 166
Brave, Ralph 146
Brennan, William 21, 132
  Dehumanizing the Vulnerable 21
Brigham, Carl 86
  A Study of American Intelligence 86
Broomall, John 118
Buck v. Bell 8, 40, 91, 93, 120, 122
Buck, Carrie 91, 116, 124, 166
Burbank, Luther 136–7
  The Training of the Human Plant
    136–7
burden, moron as 119, 123, 138
Burleigh, Michael 66, 71, 137, 147
  Death and Deliverance 71
Butler, Amos 36, 69
Byers, Joseph 35

Campbell, Clarence 90
cancer or tumor, moron as 29, 33–4
Carlson, Elof 116, 168
    Unfit, The 116
carrier or vessel, moron as 35–6, 40, 46,
    141
castration *see* eugenic control methods
    sterilization
Chamberlain, Houston Stewart 10, 107
changelings 59
Chatterton-Hill, George 30
    Heredity and Selection in Society 30
Christianity, eugenics and 109–11, 122,
    124–5
Churchill, Winston 120
civil liberties or human rights, restriction
    of
    altruism metaphor and 107, 118
    animal metaphor and 69, 72
    war metaphor and 83–5, 88, 99
Clark, L. Pierce 141
Cogdell, Christina 9, 139–42
    Eugenic Design 9, 139–42
Cohn, Norman 84
Cole, Leon 39, 123, 140, 146
Committee on Cooperation with
    Clergymen 111
Congressional Record 22
conservation, eugenics and 140–41
contagion, virus and pollution, moron as
    source of 34–7, 45–6, 141–2, 165
criminal, moron as 67, 93–4, 118, 146,
    163
Currell, Susan 9

Darré, Richard 137
Darwin, Charles 59, 96
Darwin, Leonard 96
Davenport, Charles 8, 34, 62–3, 66–8,
    70, 89–90, 97, 111, 143, 161, 164
Davenport, Gertrude 63, 115
Davis, James 98
deafness, eugenics and 165–6
defective delinquent 93–4
defectives or degenerates 6, 163
degeneration 59, 68, 85, 96, 110, 125,
    140

DeGobineau, Arthur 10, 56, 107
dehumanization 2, 12, 21, 56, 161
democracy, eugenics and 91–3
Der Sturmer 84
Deutsch, Nathanial 39, 151
DeVilbiss, Lydia 114
De Vos, George 20
disability 160, 163–70
    bioethics and 161
    see also genetics or heredity,
        eugenics and
    eugenics and 163–5
    identity and 22, 152
diseased entity, moron as 36–40, 42
Dix, Dorothea 60
Dodge, Earnest 89
Down syndrome 170
duBois, Page 57
Dudziak, Mary 91, 122
Dugdale, Robert 115, 163

East, Edward 142
efficiency movement, eugenics and
    139–40, 148
Elks, Martin 72
Emerson, Haven 140
enemy force, moron as 85–7, 93, 95, 99
English, Daylanne 10, 146
Erikson, Erik 54
Estabrook, Arthur 69
eugenic control methods
    birth control 8, 111, 144–5, 170
    euthanasia 5, 42–3, 70–2, 74, 87, 97,
        112–13, 122–3
    immigration control 8–9, 41, 88, 95,
        98
    incentive provision 8, 145, 150–1
    institutionalization 8, 40, 71, 93–4,
        118–19, 148, 165
    marriage restriction 8, 112, 136, 146
    sterilization 8, 40–1, 97, 115–16,
        120–2, 148, 150, 165–6, 169–70
    see also Nazi eugenics
eugenic family studies 7–8, 135, 137, 146
    see also Bilder Clan, Family of Sam
        Sixty, Juke family, Kallikak family,
        Piney family, Tribe of Ishmael

Eugenical News 111
eugenicist defined 5
Eugenics 138
eugenics defined 2–6
Eugenics Catechism 111
Eugenics Record Office 8, 42, 89, 138
euthanasia *see* eugenic control methods
euthenics 7, 44, 87, 117, 136, 164
evil or sinner, moron as 113–14
  see also sexually immoral, moron as
evolution, eugenics and 3, 57, 66–8, 85,
  89, 109, 124, 141, 167
experimental subject, moron as 74,
  145–6

Fairchild, Henry 31
Family of Sam Sixty 93
  see also eugenic family studies
feeble-mindedness 1, 6–7, 164–5
feral children 60
Fernald, Walter 37, 42, 93–4, 116
Fernald radiation studies 74
  see also experimental subject, moron as
Fernald School 46
filth, moron and 34, 37–8
First National Conference on Race
  Betterment 140
Fisher, Irving 111
fitter families contests 10, 111
  see also better babies contests
flood metaphor 85, 98, 111
foreign entity, moron as 44, 98
Foucault, Michel 21, 60
Frankle, Charles 124
Frazer, Elizabeth 98
'freak' shows 59, 145–6, 163
Freudian psychotherapy 165
Friedlander, Henry 149

Gallagher, Hugh Gregory 167
Galton, Sir Francis 2, 7, 58, 64, 67–8, 108
Gamble, Clarence 41
genetics or heredity, eugenics and 3, 5–6,
  113, 145, 163–6
  contemporary bioethics, eugenics and
  3, 6, 124, 161, 168–70
germ plasm 40, 68, 114, 141–2, 148

Goddard, Henry 35–6, 63–5, 87, 93, 115,
  118, 120, 123, 137, 163–4, 166
Goffman, Erving 21
Goldhagen, Daniel 133
Golden Rule, the 110
Goodey, C.F. 59
Gosney, E.S. 40–1, 115, 121
Gould, Steven Jay 18–19, 73, 147, 162
  Dinosaur in a Haystack 18
  Mismeasure of Man, The 147
Grant, Madison 141, 161
Great Chain of Being 56–7, 66, 73, 106,
  124, 132
Great Depression, eugenics and 9, 88,
  149
Guett, Arthur 43
Guyer, Michael 36, 63, 86, 90, 92, 96, 98,
  116, 135, 143
  Being Well-Born 90

Hadamar asylum 107
Hadden, Walter 70, 110
Haeckel, Ernst 57
Hartheim asylum 149
Haiseldon, Harry 40, 42, 65, 67, 69, 72,
  87, 90, 112–13, 122, 143
Hall, Prescott 95
Hasian, Marouf 3–4, 116, 167
  *The Rhetoric of Eugenics in Anglo-
  American Thought* 167
heredity, *see* genetics or heredity,
  eugenics and
Himmler, Heinrich 137, 162
Hitler, Adolf 4, 10–11, 42–3, 71, 89, 124,
  133, 137
  Mein Kampf 10, 42
Hoche, Alfred 65, 71, 120, 143
Holmes, Judge Oliver Wendell 91
Holmes, S.J. 93
Hooton, Earnest A. 33, 39, 68, 92, 97,
  111
Horsman, Reginald 57
hubris, eugenics as 109, 123
Human Genome Project 124, 168
  see also genetics or heredity, eugenics
  and
Humphrey, Seth 92

Huntington, Ellsworth 33, 112–13, 122,
    136, 139
  The Builders of America 136
  Tomorrow's Children 33

identification, dehumanizing metaphors
    and 21–2, 132, 152
idiot 6, 35, 64–5, 88, 118, 124
imbecile 6, 35, 66, 86, 93, 116
immigration *see* eugenic control methods
immigration restriction movement 8–9,
    41, 44–5, 88, 95, 98, 134
immoral, moron as
  see sexually immoral, moron as
imperialism 107
incentive provision *see* eugenic control
    methods
incubus, moron as 114
indigestible food, organism metaphor
    and 30–1, 41
infanticide, eugenics and 143, 166
  see also Bollinger Baby
insanity *see* mental illness, eugenics and
insensitive being, moron as, 64–5
instinctual or non-rational being, moron
    as 60, 62–3
institutionalization *see* eugenic control
    methods
intelligence, eugenics and 40, 61–2,
    65–7, 73–4, 93, 139
  see also instinctual or non-rational
    being, moron as
intelligence testing 7, 9, 35, 64–5, 73, 86,
    92, 162, 164–6

Jackobson, Dr. Arthur 66
Jackson, Mark 146
  The Borderland of Imbecility 146
Jacobson v. Massachusetts 40
Jesus, religious metaphor and 110–11,
    119, 122
Johnson, Alexander 86, 119, 136
Johnson, Roswell Hill 116
Johnstone, E.R. 93, 120
Journal of Heredity 89, 92
Juke family 8, 70, 115, 142, 148, 163
  see also eugenic family studies

Kallikak, Deborah 37, 116, 120
Kallikak family 8, 35–6, 38, 40, 64–5, 86,
    115, 117, 137, 147, 152
  see also eugenic family studies
Kallikak, Martin 36, 115, 137
Keen, Sam 20, 55, 84, 151
  Faces of the Enemy 84
Keene, George 67, 138
Kellogg, John Harvey 61, 68
Keller, Helen 166
Kempton, J.H. 148
Kennedy, Foster 70, 112
Kerlin, Isaac 120
Kite, Elizabeth 36, 38–9, 65, 69
Klein, Alfons 107–8
Kline, Wendy 5–6, 88, 116, 144
  Building a Better Race 5
Knight, George 69, 88
Kostir, Mary 70, 93

Le Bourdais, D.M. 121
Lakoff, George 19, 23–4
Lane, Harlan 60
Laughlin, Harry 8–9, 42, 88, 96, 111,
    136, 161
Le Chêne, Evelyn 134
Lennox, William G. 122
lethal selection, *see* eugenic control
    methods, euthanasia
Levin, Murray B. 24–30
Levine, Donald 29
liability or resource drain, moron as 142,
    147–8, 150
Lifton, Robert 71
Linnaeus, Carolus 56, 106
Little, C.C. 148
Livneh, Hanoch 46
Lombroso, Cesare 57–8, 64, 67, 93
Lovejoy, Arthur 56, 107

MacMurchy, Helen 36, 113, 138
Mallon, Mary (Typhoid Mary) 31
Malthus, Thomas 91, 95, 147
manifest destiny 107, 118
marginalization 2, 5, 11, 19–20, 25,
    72
marriage certificates 112

marriage restriction *see* eugenic control methods
maternal impressions 60–1, 147
masturbation 116
Maudsley, Henry 58
Maxwell, Ann 146
Picture Imperfect 146
McCulloch, Oscar 39
McDougall, William 150
McKim, W. Duncan 61, 122
medical experimentation *see* experimental subject, moron as
Menchen, H.L. 38, 65, 150
'Utopia by Sterilization' 150
Mendel's laws of inheritance 7, 33, 36, 164–5
see also genetics or heredity, eugenics and
menial laborer, moron as 138–9, 140–2
mental illness or insanity, eugenics and 8, 11, 59–60, 67, 71, 121, 124, 163, 165
metaphors
described 2, 18–20
marginalized groups and 20–2, 161
public policy and 19–24, 161
miscegenation 8, 10, 35, 67, 85, 106–7, 114–16, 134
missing link, moron as 59
mongrel, moron as 67
monkey or ape, moron as 58–60, 62, 66–8
moral imbecile 93–4, 163
morons 6–7, 35, 164–6
creation of word 1, 26, 135
soldiers and 86, 89–91, 142–3
motion pictures or films, eugenics and 71, 122–3, 147
Mott, Alice 58, 64
Murdoch, J.M. 86
Musolff, Andreas 29, 43
Metaphors and Political Discourse 29

Nazi eugenics 4, 10–11, 42–3, 71, 73, 85, 90, 136–7, 145, 147, 149
blood and soil program 137

horticulture metaphor and 137
organism metaphor and 32, 42–3
race hygiene 1, 4, 10, 32, 42–3
sterilization program 10–11, 89
T-4 euthanasia program 5, 11, 43, 89, 122–3, 143, 147, 149
women and 145
see also Himmler, Heinrich; Hitler, Adolf
negative eugenics 7, 97
new religion, eugenics as 108–9
Nies, Betty 35
Nietzsche, Friedrich 124–5
Thus Spoke Zarathustra 125
Noël, Lise 21–2, 30, 132
Norplant 170
Noyes, John Humphrey 108–9

object of production, moron as 139–42
Olby, Robert 106
Olson, Judge Harry 69, 94
Oneida Community 108–9

parasite, moron as 39–40, 62, 149, 162
parens patriae 119
Patterns of Prejudice 43
pauper, moron as 39, 120, 147, 163, 170
Pearl, Raymond 69
penetration or ingestion, organism metaphor and 30–1, 46
perfectionist communities 108–9
Pernick, Martin 40, 42, 65, 67, 72, 122, 147
Black Stork, the 122, 147
perpetual child, moron as 118, 124
philanthropy, eugenicists' view of 39, 108, 114
photography, eugenics and 38, 133, 146–7
Pinel, Phillipe 60
Piney family 36, 69
see also eugenic family studies
plague, moron as 34–5
poison, moron as 35, 37
polygenesis 106
Popenoe, Paul 115–16, 121, 150
positive eugenics 7, 10, 90, 139, 144

Powlison, Charles 63
Proctor, Robert 89–90
Progressive movement 9, 44, 87, 112,
    162, 164–5
prostitute, moron as
    see sexually immoral, moron as
pruning, object metaphor and 137
public health movement, eugenics and
    9, 25, 33, 36, 39, 40–3, 44–5, 109,
    124, 162

quarantine, organism metaphor and 32,
    35–6, 40

race suicide 10, 45, 68, 90–1, 95–6, 145,
    147
racial anthropology 10, 107, 134
racial hierarchy see species hierarchy
Rafter, Nicole 38–9, 69, 135
    White Trash 38
Reader's Digest 34
Recapitulation 67–8
registration of feeble-minded 42, 89
reification of metaphors 45–6, 55,
    162
religious leaders, eugenics and 111–12
religious symbols, movement use of 105,
    111, 122
Risley, S.D. 116
Ritvo, Harriet 73
Rivera, Geraldo 74
Robie, Dr. Theodore 114
Robinson, Caroline 39, 87
Roosevelt, Theodore 90, 141, 144
Rosen, Christine 111–12
    Preaching Eugenics 111
Ryan, Patrick 170

Sanborn, Bigelow 119
Sanger, Margaret 8–9, 66, 138, 144–5,
    148
Sax, Boria 72
Schön, Donald 18, 23
Schwartz, Karl 97, 113, 140
self-defense, war metaphor and 99
self-improvement, eugenics and 9,
    162

sexually immoral, moron as 36–7, 96,
    114–15, 122, 124, 143, 163
Sherbon, Francis 33–4, 39
Shick, Mary 121
Shipley, Maynard 71
Singer, Peter 74
Smith, J. David 54, 117
social Darwinism 30, 91, 107, 109, 116,
    141
social purity movement 9, 117
Sontag, Susan 18, 44
Southard, D.D. 138
species hierarchy 65–7, 72–4, 132
speciesism 74
Spencer, Herbert 30, 32
    Social Statics 32
Spiro, Jonathon 141
sterilization see eugenic control methods
Stern, Leon 33, 61
Stoddard, Lothrop 33–4, 42, 66, 70, 92,
    95–7, 117, 142, 150
    Rising Tide of Color 95
stream metaphor 141–2
Suárez-Orozco, Marcelo 20
sub-human, primitive or atavistic being,
    moron as 38, 66–71, 73–4
Sumner, Walter 112
superman, the 125
Survey 136, 141
Sylva, Kathryn 146
Szasz, Thomas 21

T-4 euthanasia program see Nazi eugenics
Taft, Jesse 123, 164
Talbot, Eugene 38, 59
taxation, eugenics and 8, 39, 82, 92,
    138–9, 148–50, 170
Tay-Sachs disease 6, 169
Taylor, Frederick 139
Third International Congress of Eugenics
    143
Third Race Betterment Conference 109,
    148
Trent, James 6, 57
Tribe of Ishmael 34, 39, 69, 116,
    152
    see also eugenic family studies

ulcer or sore, moron as 33, 43
unit-trait theory 164

valueless or worthless object, moron as
    142–3, 147, 162
venereal disease 9, 36–8, 116–7, 122
Victor, the 'Wild Boy of Aveyron' 60
Vogt, Carl 59
von Maltitz, Horst 54

Walker, General F.A. 95–6
war, eugenics and 87, 89–91, 100, 141
Ward, Robert 33, 41
Warthin, Alfred Scott 109, 113
waste product, moron as 31, 132,
    137
weed or bad crop, moron as 110, 135–9,
    142
Weindling, Paul 42, 121
Weingartner, James 135
Weiss, Feri 88
    Seive, The 88

welfare, eugenicists and 94, 147, 170
Wells, Kate 113
Whetham, Catherine 111
Whetham, William 111
Whitney, E.A. 121, 148
Whitney, Leon 61, 109–10, 112–13, 122,
    136, 139, 147, 150
Wiggam, Albert 34, 68, 86, 107, 109–10,
    120–1
    New Decalogue of Science, The 111
Willowbrook 45, 74
Willowbrook hepatitis study 74
Wolfensberger, Wolf 20, 74, 118, 124
women, eugenicists and 87, 113–15,
    121–2, 143–5
    see also sexually immoral, moron as
Wright, A.O. 63, 163

Yukins, Elizabeth 37, 137, 144

Zenderland, Leila 118, 120
Zuckier, Henri 25

9 781784 991074